Neuroimaging in Ophthalmology

Ophthalmology Monographs

A *series published by* Oxford *University Press in cooperation*
with the American Academy of Ophthalmology

Series Editor: Richard K. Parrish, II, MD, Bascom Palmer Eye Institute

American Academy of Ophthalmology Clinical Education Secretariat:
Louis B. Cantor, MD, Indiana University School of Medicine
Gregory L. Skuta, MD, Dean A. McGee Eye Institute

NEUROIMAGING IN OPHTHALMOLOGY

Second Edition

Michael C. Johnson, MD, FRCSC
Bruno A. Policeni, MD
Andrew G. Lee, MD
Wendy R. K. Smoker, MD, FACR

Published by Oxford University Press
in cooperation with
the American Academy of Ophthalmology

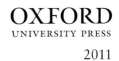

OXFORD
UNIVERSITY PRESS
2011

OXFORD

UNIVERSITY PRESS

Oxford University Press, Inc., publishes works that further
Oxford University's objective of excellence
in research, scholarship, and education.

Oxford New York
Auckland Cape Town Dar es Salaam Hong Kong Karachi
Kuala Lumpur Madrid Melbourne Mexico City Nairobi
New Delhi Shanghai Taipei Toronto

With offices in
Argentina Austria Brazil Chile Czech Republic France Greece
Guatemala Hungary Italy Japan Poland Portugal Singapore
South Korea Switzerland Thailand Turkey Ukraine Vietnam

Published by Oxford University Press, Inc.
198 Madison Avenue, New York, New York 10016
www.oup.com

Oxford is a registered trademark of Oxford University Press

Library of Congress Cataloging-in-Publication Data

Neuroimaging in ophthalmology / Michael C. Johnson ... [et al.].—2nd ed.
p. ; cm.—(Ophthalmology monographs ; 6)
Rev. ed. of: Magnetic resonance imaging and computed tomography / Jonathan D. Wirtschafter,
Eric L. Berman, Carolyn S. McDonald. c1992.
Includes bibliographical references.
ISBN 978-0-19-538161-0
1. Eye—Magnetic resonance imaging—Atlases. 2. Eye—Tomography—Atlases. 3. Visual pathways—Magnetic
resonance imaging—Atlases. 4. Visual pathways—Tomography—Atlases. I. Johnson, Michael C. (Michael Curtis),
1975– II. Wirtschafter, Jonathan Dine, 1935– Magnetic resonance imaging and computed tomography. III. Series:
Ophthalmology monographs ; 6.
[DNLM: 1. Eye Diseases—diagnosis—Atlases. 2. Eye—anatomy & histology—Atlases. 3. Magnetic Resonance
Imaging—methods—Atlases. 4. Tomography, X-Ray Computed—methods—Atlases. W1 OP372L v.6 2010 / WW 17
N494 2010]
QM511.W55 2010
617.7'1548—dc22
2010002566

9 8 7 6 5 4 3 2 1

Printed in China

Legal Notice

The American Academy of Ophthalmology provides the opportunity for material to be presented for educational purposes only. The material represents the approach, ideas, statements, or opinion of the authors, not necessarily the only or best method or procedure in every case, nor the position of the Academy. Unless specifically stated otherwise, the opinions expressed and statements made by various authors in this monograph reflect the authors' observations and do not imply endorsement by the Academy. The material is not intended to replace a physician's own judgment or to give specific advice for case management. The Academy does not endorse any of the products or companies, if any, mentioned in this monograph.

Some material on recent developments may include information on drug or device applications that are not considered community standard, that reflect indications not included in approved FDA labeling, or that are approved for use only in restricted research settings. This information is provided as education only so physicians may be aware of alternative methods of the practice of medicine, and should not be considered endorsement, promotion, or in any way encouragement to use such applications. The FDA has stated that it is the responsibility of the physician to determine the FDA status of each drug or device he or she wishes to use in clinical practice, and to use these products with appropriate patient consent and in compliance with applicable law.

The Academy and Oxford University Press (OUP) do not make any warranties as to the accuracy, adequacy, or completeness of any material presented here, which is provided on an "as is" basis. The Academy and OUP are not liable to anyone for any errors, inaccuracies, or omissions obtained here. The Academy specifically disclaims any and all liability for injury or other damages of any kind for any and all claims that may arise out of the use of any practice, technique, or drug described in any material by any author, whether such claims are asserted by a physician or any other person.

DISCLOSURE STATEMENT

Unless otherwise noted below, each author states that he or she has no significant financial interest or other relationship with the manufacturer of any commercial product discussed in the chapters that he or she contributed to this publication or with the manufacturer of any competing commercial product.

Preface

Neuroimaging and orbital imaging using computed tomography (CT) and magnetic resonance imaging (MRI) techniques have revolutionized the evaluation, management, and treatment of orbital and neuro-ophthalmic disorders. Despite the increased resolution of these imaging studies, it is critical for the diagnosing clinician/ordering physician and the interpreting radiologist to communicate with one another clearly and explicitly about the relevant topographical anatomy, to confirm the localizing value of the clinical findings, to generate a compatible differential diagnosis, and, most important, to correlate the clinical findings with the radiographic findings (i.e., "clinical correlation required").

It is our hope that this revision of the original AAO neuroimaging monograph will assist clinicians in understanding the mechanics of the imaging techniques (i.e., CT and MRI), the indications and contraindications for specific imaging, and the clinicoradiologic correlation of specific neuro-ophthalmic or orbital presentations.

The authors of the current edition wish to acknowledge and thank the authors of the first edition (Dr. Eric Berman, Dr. Jonathan Wirtschafter,* and Dr. Carolyn Johnson) for their work, which served as the basis for this revision. We would also like to acknowledge Dr. Daniel Thedens, PhD, for his work in reviewing the physics section of this monograph.

We have tried to update, rather than completely replace, the content of the original version, especially in the areas of neuroimaging that have not changed significantly over time. To update the monograph, a literature review was performed by the current authors using a systematic English-language MEDLINE search (1994–2008) limited to articles with relevance to neuro-ophthalmic and orbital imaging.

The new information in this monograph includes the following: 1) an update on the basic mechanics, indications, and contraindications for cranial and orbital CT and MRI, 2) the indications and contraindications for intravenous contrast (e.g., iodinated contrast for CT and gadolinium contrast for MRI), and 3) the basics of specific MR sequences and specific techniques (e.g., CT/MR angiography and venography). Because of space limitations, detailed discussion of the functional imaging techniques such as functional MRI (fMRI), positron emission tomography (PET) scanning, and single-photon emission computed tomography (SPECT) are not included in this monograph.

In the original version of this monograph, Chapter 1 provided a nonmathematical introduction to the physics of imaging. We have tried to simplify this portion of the original text and provide a more concise and clinically meaningful context for the basics of the imaging techniques for the targeted audience of this monograph. The basic physics for the imaging studies might help the reader better understand CT and MRI such that studies are ordered and interpreted more precisely and efficiently. Chapters 1 through 3 are intended to provide a basic framework for the normal and pathologic radiologic findings seen in various disease entities of interest to the ophthalmologist. Chapter 4, the last section of the monograph, provides the reader with guidelines for ordering the proper imaging study and provides specific pathologic examples of interest to the ophthalmologist.

Michael C. Johnson, MD, FRCSC
Bruno A. Policeni, MD
Andrew G. Lee, MD
Wendy R. K. Smoker, MD, FACR
*Dr. Wirtschafter is deceased.

Contents

Introduction

Ophthalmologists are often the first clinicians to evaluate the patient harboring an underlying intraorbital or intracranial structural lesion. The prescribing (i.e., physician ordering the imaging study) ophthalmologist must therefore understand the basic mechanics, indications, and contraindications for the available orbital and neuroimaging studies (e.g., computed tomography [CT] and magnetic resonance imaging [MRI]), as well as the special studies that may be necessary to fully evaluate the suspected pathology. In addition, the prescribing physician must communicate the imaging question and provide relevant clinical information to the interpreting physician (i.e., radiologist) to obtain the best imaging interpretation. Since the publication of the original edition of this monograph, newer techniques and special sequences have improved the ability to detect pathology in the orbit and brain of interest to the ophthalmologist. Table A-1 lists the clinical scenarios for which an imaging study might be ordered by an ophthalmologist.

In this second version of the monograph, we update the original content and summarize the recent neuroradiologic literature on the various modalities applicable to CT and MRI for ophthalmology. The mainstays for orbital and neuroimaging are conventional radiography (e.g., skull film), CT, and MRI. Although catheter angiography was considered a "mainstay" in the past, this has now been largely replaced by CT angiography (CTA) and MR angiography (MRA). The x-ray has been known since the time of Roentgen, for which he received a Nobel Prize. The role of the traditional skull or orbital radiograph has been supplanted in the modern era by current CT and MR techniques, and we will not discuss in detail the radiograph beyond its historical uses. At our institutions, we still use the skull radiograph in a limited role to prescreen patients with a history or suspicion for metallic foreign body prior to MR studies. As a general rule, patients who

Table A-1. Common Clinical Scenarios for Which an Imaging Study Might Be Prescribed by an Ophthalmologist

1. Unilateral or bilateral visual loss (e.g., transient visual loss [amaurosis fugax], unilateral or bilateral optic neuropathy, junctional scotoma, bitemporal hemianopsia, homonymous hemianopsia, cortical blindness, or combinations of these)
2. Efferent neurogenic pupillary defects (e.g., anisocoria due to Horner syndrome or third nerve palsy)
3. Afferent pupillary defects (e.g., relative afferent papillary defect or light-near dissociation of the pupils)
4. Proptosis (e.g., thyroid eye disease, orbital tumors, idiopathic orbital inflammation [i.e., orbital pseudotumor], orbital cellulitis, or carotid-cavernous fistula) or enophthalmos [i.e., orbital fracture])
5. Diplopia or external ophthalmoplegia
6. Eye lid abnormalities (e.g., lid retraction, lid lag, ptosis, or palpable orbital-lid lesion)
7. Oscillopsia (e.g., nystagmus)
8. Ophthalmoscopic abnormalities suggesting an orbital or intracranial lesion (e.g., papilledema, optic atrophy, optic nerve hypoplasia, optic disc head drusen, or choroidal folds)
9. Ocular or orbital trauma (e.g., intraocular/intraorbital foreign body or suspected fracture)

*In this monograph, we have elected to not include the neuroimaging evaluation of isolated headache, facial pain, or other non–neuro-ophthalmic or nonorbital indications for neuroimaging.

have an indication for orbital imaging should undergo a CT or MR study, if not contraindicated, as these both have improved bone or soft tissue resolution over conventional plain films.

We have chosen to emphasize vascular imaging advances (e.g., MRA, CTA, MR venography [MRV], and CT venography [CTV]) and specific MR sequences (e.g., fat suppression, fluid attenuation inversion recovery [FLAIR], gradient recall echo imaging [GRE], diffusion-weighted imaging [DWI], perfusion-weighted imaging [PWI], and dynamic perfusion CT [PCT]). The goal of the monograph is to reinforce the critical importance of accurate, complete, and timely communication of the clinical findings, the differential diagnosis, and the presumptive topographical location of the suspected lesion from the prescribing ophthalmologist to the interpreting radiologist in order to perform the optimal imaging study and to ultimately receive the best interpretation. We provide tables to summarize the indications and best imaging recommendations for specific ophthalmic entities, and we have collected a number of examples of specific radiographic pathology to illustrate the relevant entities.

About the Authors

Michael C. Johnson, MD, FRCSC is an assistant professor in the department of ophthalmology at the University of Alberta, Edmonton, Alberta, Canada.

Bruno Policeni, MD, is a clinical assistant professor of diagnostic radiology—neuroradiology, University of Iowa.

Andrew G. Lee, MD is chair of the department of ophthalmology at The Methodist Hospital in Houston, Texas, and is professor of ophthalmology in neurology and neurological surgery at Weill Cornell Medical College. Dr. Lee serves on the Editorial Board of 12 journals including the *American Journal of Ophthalmology*, the *Canadian Journal of Ophthalmology*, and *Eye* and he has published over 270 peer-reviewed articles, 40 book chapters, and 3 full textbooks in ophthalmology.

Wendy K. Smoker, MD, FACR is a professor of radiology, neurology, and neurosurgery, and division director of neuroradiology at the University of Iowa Hospitals and Clinics. Dr. Smoker has served on the Editorial Board of multiple radiology journals, previously a deputy editor of *Radiology*. She has authored or coauthored 144 scientific publications, presented 282 invited lectures, and authored or co-authored 47 book chapters.

1

Magnetic Resonance Imaging

The demonstration of human anatomy using the techniques of magnetic resonance (MR) was first accomplished by a team led by Sir Peter Mansfield at the University of Nottingham in 1976. This accomplishment rests on a broadly based body of knowledge and techniques that encompasses much of modern physics. The scientific foundation involves notions of atomic and molecular structure and the concept of nuclear MR (NMR). First observed in the late 1940s, the actual phenomenon of NMR could be produced in uniform, bulk materials contained in test tubes or similar chambers. In 1973, Paul C. Lauterbur suggested that magnetic field gradients could encode position-dependent imaging information. For their work on MR techniques, in 2003 Lauterbur and Mansfield received the Nobel Prize (in Physiology or Medicine), as Wilhelm Conrad Röntgen (1901 Nobel Prize in Physics) and Godfrey N. Hounsfield (1979 Nobel Prize in Physiology and Medicine) had before them.

1-1 PHYSICAL PRINCIPLES

Despite the technical complexity of MR imaging (MRI), ophthalmologists will be encouraged to know that the physics of MR can be more easily understood by emphasizing models that are analogous to those used for explaining the physics of light; however, if you prefer to skip the denser part of MRI physics, go to Section 1-7.

Some phenomena of light can best be described by classic wave theory, while other phenomena of light are best illustrated by quantum particle theory, even though the two approaches may have apparent contradictions. Similarly, the physics of MRI can sometimes best be understood with a quantum-mechanical model, in which each proton can be in either one of two states (parallel or antiparallel), or with a classic mechanical model, in which the net magnetic moment vector of all protons can be located with regard to a three-dimensional frame of reference. This three-dimensional frame of reference may be considered either as stationary, with its x and y axes fixed and perpendicular to the main (static) magnetic field (the laboratory frame of reference), or as rotating, with its x and y axes rotating in synchrony with the precessing protons (the rotating frame of reference).

MRI is based on the principle that the nuclei of certain atoms become polarized or aligned (display magnetic moments) when placed in a static magnetic field (Figure 1-1). This magnetic property is present only if the nucleus contains an odd number of protons and/or neutrons. In particular, it is the odd number of protons in the nuclei of hydrogen (^{1}H), sodium (^{23}Na), and phosphorus (^{31}P) that is responsible for the magnetic moments in human tissues. This realignment is

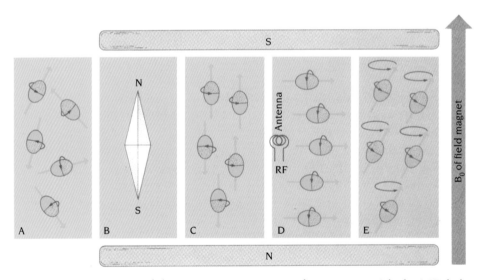

Figure 1-1. Comparison of the magnetic properties of a compass with the MR behavior of protons in several states. (A) No magnet: in the absence of a magnetic field, the protons are randomly aligned. (B) Compass needle in magnetic field: the compass needle aligns with the magnet but can point in only one direction. (C) In the main magnetic field: the magnetized protons are "flipped" to align with the magnetic field, B_0, but may align parallel or antiparallel to the applied magnetic field. More protons align with the field than against it. The possibility of two orientations for the protons differs from the one orientation allowed for the compass needle. (D) Immediately after application of a 90° RF pulse: the imposition of a 90° RF pulse by an antenna (diagrammed as a coil) causes all the protons that contributed to the net magnetic vector to flip in one direction in the transverse plans, where they all precess in phase. (E) Partial longitudinal relaxation and precession: after the end of a 90° RF burst, the protons relax toward the longitudinal axis and are seen precessing around that axis. A similar result occurs when the RF pulse is shorter than a pulse required for a 90° displacement. Such a pulse is said to tilt the protons and is used in various imaging sequences.

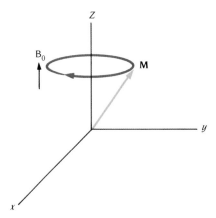

Figure 1-2. The nuclear magnetization vector **M** rotates at the Larmor frequency around the main magnetic field vector B_0, which is defined as oriented in the z axis. M rotates in the clockwise direction (from *y* to *x*) as viewed from above at the Larmor frequency. The MRI signal obtained from the protons in each voxel must be detected and processed to obtain useful information.

a statistical phenomenon, for not all nuclei will be identically realigned. When the magnetic field (designated as B_0) is activated, all of the atomic nuclei will be affected. However, a slightly smaller fraction (a few parts per million) of the nuclei will align against B_0 than with it, creating a net magnetic vector in the longitudinal direction of the magnetic field, designated the *z* axis (Figure 1-2). The behavior of hydrogen nuclei (protons) in a magnetic field can be compared and contrasted to that of a compass. The compass needle always points in one direction, but protons can align either parallel or antiparallel to the magnetic field. The protons aligned in the parallel direction are at a lower energy level than those aligned in the antiparallel direction. A quantum of energy must be absorbed by a proton oriented in the parallel direction for it to be transformed into a proton oriented in the antiparallel direction. Conversely, a proton oriented in the antiparallel direction must lose a quantum of energy to be transformed to a parallel orientation.

Transformations between parallel and antiparallel orientations can occur if the proton gains or emits energy by gaining or emitting one photon (as a radiofrequency [RF] wave) of the correct energy. Moreover, a proton in an antiparallel orientation can be struck by one photon and emit two photons, resulting in an energy loss sufficient to transform the proton to a parallel orientation. Low-strength magnets cause nearly equal numbers of protons to align in each direction, but as the magnetic field strength is increased, the energy difference between the two states also increases and more of the magnetic dipoles of the individual protons tend to align in the lowest energy state parallel to the main magnetic field. This creates a net magnetic vector parallel to the direction of the magnet.

For each isotope that possesses a nuclear magnetic moment (e.g., ^{1}H or ^{31}P), there is a characteristic resonant frequency (Larmor frequency) at which it absorbs energy. The Larmor frequency is related to intrinsic properties of that element and is directly proportional to the strength of the static magnetic field (measured in Tesla, abbreviated T). Thus, application of an RF wave of resonant frequency equal to the Larmor frequency provides the energy that will produce a realignment of the magnetic vector. This application of energy is called *excitation*. This energy is re-emitted from the protons over time through a process known as *relaxation*. During relaxation, the torque of the static magnetic field exerted on the magnetic moment of the protons causes them to exhibit a type of movement called *precession*: the protons behave like small tops spinning around the axis of the magnetic field vector (see Figure 1-1). We are familiar with the force of gravity that causes the precession of a spinning top or gyroscope; when the device falls over, relaxation is completed. In the case of MRI, the magnetic force causes complete relaxation when all of the protons are realigned with the main magnetic field. Relaxation is the process whereby the absorbed energy is redistributed among the aligned protons (there is also some loss to the neighboring nuclei). Relaxation releases energy at the Larmor frequency and this energy can be detected with an antenna, often the same antenna that was used to excite the protons.

1-2 EXTRACTION OF SPATIAL INFORMATION

Once the protons are in an aligned equilibrium orientation, it becomes possible to use a burst of electromagnetic energy to manipulate the protons and produce clinically useful information. The imposition of the main magnetic field is somewhat analogous to installing the strings on a musical instrument and then applying tension to them (tuning). The tuning is accomplished by the gradient magnetic field. The plucking of the proton "strings" is done with a short pulse or burst of RF whose magnetic field is perpendicular to the static magnetic field. This RF pulse provides energy that is absorbed by the protons and brings them to a more excited state, which changes the direction of their magnetic vectors. The length and amplitude of the pulse can be varied to control the degree of change in the magnetic vector. The RF bursts are most commonly designated as 90° or 180° pulses. The resultant movements of the protons can be called flips or tilts (see Figure 1-1). When the net magnetic vector is flipped 90° to the longitudinal axis (z), it is located in the transverse (x,y) plane.

In current clinical practice, only protons are used to produce MRI scans, because protons are abundant in the human body as water and the signal from hydrogen protons is easily detected. Most of the energy re-emitted by the protons in the tissue is absorbed within the tissue, but a small fraction of the energy is absorbed by the antenna receiver coil. The detected signal is proportional to the spin density—the number of nuclear magnetic moments per unit volume. The signal is received by an antenna arranged to detect precession of the magnetic dipole of protons only while they remain aligned in the transverse plane. When a signal is recorded as described earlier, it is described as a measurement of free induction decay (FID). The longitudinal decay of each proton within the slice is somewhat analogous to that of each atom within a volume of unstable isotopes of one element, in that it behaves independently with its own timing. FID signals are not used clinically because their half-lives are not sufficiently long to allow the application of gradients necessary to localize the signals and generate an image in human patients. The pulse sequences that are used to produce clinically useful signals are discussed in Sections 1-7 to 1-12. The emitted signals are transformed by the computer into an image by a mathematical process called two- or three-dimensional Fourier transformation. This produces the familiar pictures seen on the monitors.

NMR was initially a technique applied to small volumes of homogeneous chemicals in a vessel within homogeneous magnetic fields. To provide useful clinical information about the inhomogeneous environments of protons within a tissue space such as the skull or orbit, it is necessary to arrange for the selective excitation of a slice of tissue with an MRI scanning device. To accomplish this, a weak inhomogeneous gradient static magnetic field is superimposed on the strong homogeneous static magnetic field supplied by the main magnet (Figure 1-3). The weak

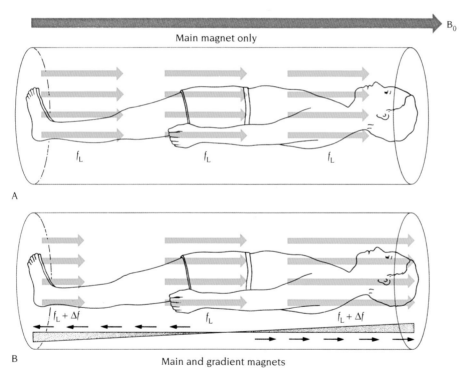

Figure 1-3. Gradient magnets can alter the local magnetic field strength (represented by arrow length) from the uniform strength imposed by the main magnet (A). When the gradient magnet field is superimposed (B), unequal field strength results. Although the progression is continuous throughout the magnetic field, the strength in only three regions is shown for simplicity. Without the gradient magnets, the resonance frequency (f) is also uniform throughout the volume, but f changes (Δf) due to the gradient. The extent of the magnetic gradient is called its bandwidth. The gradient magnet tunes the system for the extraction of spatial information. For example, only the slice containing the head would be selected by an RF pulse of $f_L + \Delta f$. (f_L = Larmor frequency induced by main magnet.)

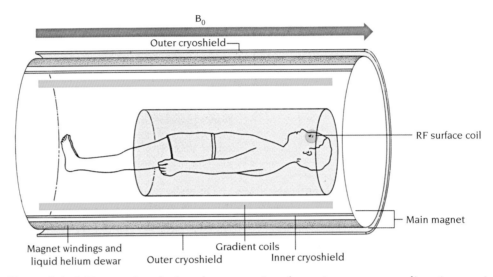

Figure 1-4. MR scanning device, demonstrating the main magnet, gradient (magnet) coils, and RF surface coils. The use of surface coils is optional. B_0, the magnetic vector of the main magnet, is in the longitudinal plane (z axis) and is shown above the device. The transverse plane (x, y axes) is perpendicular to the longitudinal axis.

magnetic field is produced by one or more accessory magnets called *gradient coils* (Figure 1-4). The inhomogeneous field varies in a predictable way with the location in the bore of the magnet. Three gradient coils are required to set up a three-dimensional imaging system.

A spatial coordinate system can be established that permits imaging of the axial, coronal, and sagittal orthogonal planes as well as oblique planes. Manipulating the gradient fields through orthogonal planes provides data for Fourier transformation and spatial reconstruction. This can be done by periodically adding y and z gradient fields to the static x gradient field.

The ability to directly obtain information in the midsagittal plane of the skull is one of the principal advantages of MRI over computed tomography (CT); however, with the new multislice CT, thin-section images with isotropic voxels (volume elements) are available and generate excellent orthogonal plane reconstructions. Once the x, y, and z gradients have been established, a change of the exciting RF is the only requirement for changing the parallel plane that is being imaged. The thickness of the parallel planes (slice thickness) is controlled by the bandwidth of the RF pulse used in the excitation (Figure 1-5).

The MRI device contains RF receiver coils, which pick up the MRI signal that will later be amplified and analyzed. Although RF receiver coils are built into the scanner, they can be temporarily disconnected and replaced by smaller coils applied directly to parts of the body surface such as the orbit. Direct application improves the signal-to-noise (S/N) ratio and thus permits acquisitions of even greater resolution. Surface coils such as head and orbit coils have specific uses for evaluating the orbit and visual system. Regardless of where the receiver coils are

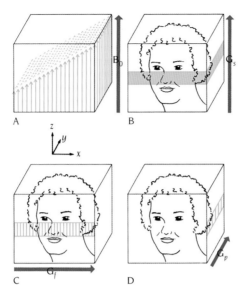

Figure 1-5. Acquisition of a single-slice, two-dimensional Fourier transform image. (A) The gradients of the magnetic field strengths within the scanned volume produced by the main and gradient magnets. The direction of the B_0 arrow indicates the main magnetic field. The direction of increasing phase difference and increasing frequency within the slice is indicated by the *arrows*. (B) The dark volume is that excited by the RF pulses within the selected frequency range: the wider the range, the greater is the slice thickness. This parameter is also designated as G_s, the slice- selection gradient. (C) The frequency-encoding gradient (Gf) is shown arbitrarily along the y axis of the transverse plane. (D) The phase- encoding gradient (G_p) is shown arbitrarily along the x axis of the transverse plane. Spatial localization within three-dimensional volumes (voxels) can be defined by the application of these gradients. The application of the x gradient while detecting the MRI signal assigns a unique frequency to each voxel according to its x coordinates. The application of a y gradient for a short period before the detection of the MRI signal assigns a unique phase to each voxel according to its y coordinates.

placed, the only useful signal that can be detected is in the transverse or x-y plane, because the dominant magnetic field arises from the main bore magnet, the location of which is fixed.

Selective excitation of protons within a single slice will result when the precession frequency of the protons within the slice is identical to that of the transmitted exciting RF (see Figure 1-5). Because the Larmor frequency is determined by the strength of the static magnetic field, it follows that the Larmor frequency will vary in a predictable manner within tissue placed in an inhomogeneous magnetic field. This inhomogeneity results when a gradient coil is turned on at the same time as the RF coil that emits the Larmor frequency. This can be used to create the selective excitation of tissue within a single slice.

Useful clinical information depends on receiving, analyzing, and displaying the analog RF signals from the excited protons. This requires collecting the data

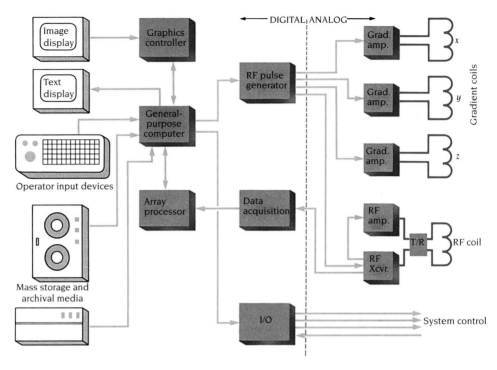

Figure 1-6. MRI scanning device. A general-purpose computer operating in a digital domain is used to control various operations in the analog domain, including the magnetic gradient coils and the RF antenna for its transmission (T) and receiver (R) functions. After the RF signal is received, it is converted from analog to digital for processing within the computer and displayed on the image display graphic device as well as the printing device. Other digital and analog interfaces are provided by the input/output (I/O) systems. (Redrawn with permission from Atlas SW. Magnetic Resonance Imaging of the Brain and Spine. New York, NY: Raven Press; 1991.)

so that they can be spatially encoded and transferred into a digital domain for further processing (Figure 1-6). There are two methods in general clinical use for spatially encoding MRI data: frequency encoding and phase encoding. *Frequency encoding* uses an antenna to record the FID frequency spectrum produced while the magnetic field gradient is switched on. The protons excited at different positions within the plane will resonate at different frequencies based on their position in the plane (Figure 1-7). The combined signal from such protons can be subjected to Fourier analysis, and projection of their relative location and intensity can be made. Thousands of repeated determinations at many angles within the plane can be made as the gradient is rotated. The gradient coil is not physically rotated but is arranged to produce the same result as the "slip ring" on a CT scanner, which does physically rotate to send and receive data.

Phase encoding also uses a magnetic field gradient to encode spatial information but in a slightly different way. Phase encoding uses the gradient to set up a difference in the amount of rotation or phase in the proton signal as a function of location

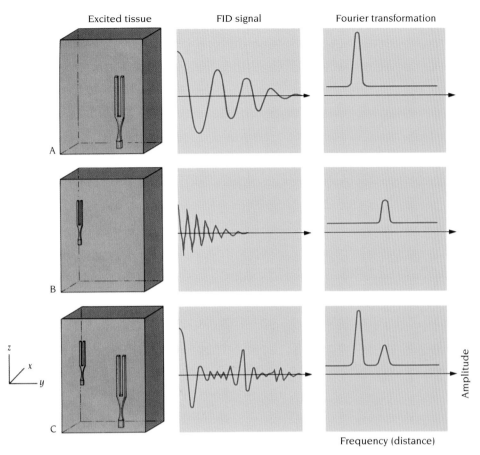

Figure 1-7. Extraction of spatial information. (A, B) Fourier transformation. (C) The sounds emitted by two tuning forks originating from the same volume merge to produce a complex waveform. Fourier transformation (*right*) identifies the source and amplitude of the two signals. RF signals emitted from relaxing protons at slightly different positions within a signal slice of tissue undergoing MRI scanning emit signals that are measured as free induction decay (FID). The protons at slightly different distances along the *y* axis emit slightly different resonant frequencies, indicated by large and small tuning forks. Frequency-encoding analysis is performed while the magnetic field gradient is switched on.

within the magnetic field. Thus, phase encoding generates a distance-dependent effect in a direction perpendicular to the frequency-encoding direction. The phase-encoding gradient is turned on after the RF pulse but before the antenna records data. Hundreds, or even thousands, of repeated determinations are obtained at different gradient strengths on each repetition. The gradient strength can be controlled by varying the current strength and direction in the coil. The combination of all of these different phase-encoding steps can be used to localize the protons in a second, or even third, direction within the magnet.

Spatial encoding is thus based on one physical principle, whether the technique used is frequency encoding or phase encoding: both measure the changes in the FID signal emitted in the presence of a gradient. The only difference is that the signal changes arising from the frequency-encoding gradient are generated during the recording of the FID signal, whereas the changes due to the phase-encoding gradient are generated before the FID signal is recorded. The signal intensity, represented on a two-dimensional projection as a pixel (picture element), is proportional to the number of protons precessing within a three-dimensional voxel (volume element) within the acquisition matrix. Repeated measurements at all projections in the transverse (x,y) plane are used to calculate the signal intensity at each pixel within the plane. The digital methods of calculation and image construction are related to those used in computed tomography.

1-3 T1 AND T2 DEFINED

Except for the main magnetic field strength, the various parameters by which MRI techniques and images are characterized are mostly related to time. T1 and T2 are time constants resulting from inherent tissue characteristics that correspond to the behavior of protons whose nuclei precess in response to applied magnetic and RFstimuli (Table 1-1). TR (repetition time), TE (time to echo), and TI (time for inversion) are time intervals selected by the personnel performing the scan and are independent of any inherent tissue characteristics. These time intervals are discussed in Section 1-4.

In MRI scanning, RF pulses of a selected energy and duration are applied to reorient the net magnetic vector from the z axis that was imposed by the static magnetic field. In most cases, the selected pulse will change the net magnetic vector by either 90° or 180°. The frequency required of the RF pulse is directly related to the magnetic field strength. With a field strength of 1.5 T, pulses of approximately 64 MHz will excite protons. These pulses are used, either singly or in combination,

Table 1-1. T1 and T2 in Various Mammalian Tissues at 1.5 T

Tissue	T1 (msec)	T2 (msec)
Muscle		
Skeletal	870	47
Heart	870	57
Liver	490	43
Spleen	560	58
Adipose	260	84
Brain		
Gray matter	920	101
White matter	790	92

Reprinted with permission from Bottomley PA, Foster TH, Argersinger RE, et al. A review of normal tissue hydrogen NMR relaxation times and relaxation mechanisms from 1–100 MHz: dependence on tissue type, NMR frequency, temperature, species, excision, and age. Med Phys. 1984;11:425–448.

to produce different pulse sequences. The term *longitudinal plane* is used for the z axis, the vector of the magnetic field prior to the onset of the RF pulse. When a suitable RF pulse is applied, all of the protons respond and become oriented 90° from the longitudinal plane (i.e., in the transverse plane). After the pulse is terminated, there will be zero magnetization from the protons in the longitudinal axis. Subsequently, the protons will slowly realign with the longitudinal magnetic field. This exponential process is called *longitudinal relaxation*. It asymptotically approaches a maximum value of 100%. By convention, the time required for proton spins comprising 63% of the vector to return to the longitudinal axis is designated T1, the longitudinal (or spin-lattice) relaxation time (Figure 1-8). This type of relaxation occurs as the stimulated protons lose their kinetic energy due to the retarding forces of neighboring nuclei in the lattice. Spin-lattice relaxation is essentially a thermal reaction, with the transfer of energy as heat from the protons to the surrounding molecular environment (lattice).

The term *transverse plane* is used for the net magnetic vector that is oriented in the *x,y* axis, located 90° from the longitudinal plane. Immediately after the 90° RF pulse is terminated, the magnetic vectors for all protons in this plane are identical. Due to slight imperfections in the static magnetic field and local variations in the magnetic moments of neighboring protons and unpaired electrons, some protons are exposed to a stronger field than others and precess at a faster rate than adjacent protons, because the rate of precession always depends on the local magnetic field experienced. The interaction of the magnetic moments of the faster-precessing with the slower-precessing protons causes loss of energy and entropy. The protons exchange their spins with their neighbors—thus, the term *spin-spin relaxation*. In a quantum-mechanical model, parallel and antiparallel protons are converted to the opposite state. This leads to a dephasing of the proton spins and causes a rapid dispersion of the magnetic vector with regard to a three-dimensional frame

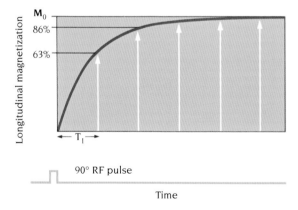

Figure 1-8. T1 relaxation. T1 is the time required for 63% of the protons comprising the net magnetic vector to return to the longitudinal plane after the cessation of a 90° RF pulse. The 63% is an arbitrary value called the time constant for an exponential process. M_0 is the maximal value and is not achieved until several multiples of T1 have passed. If the repetition time (TR) is equal to T1, longitudinal remagnetization will not have time to be fully completed.

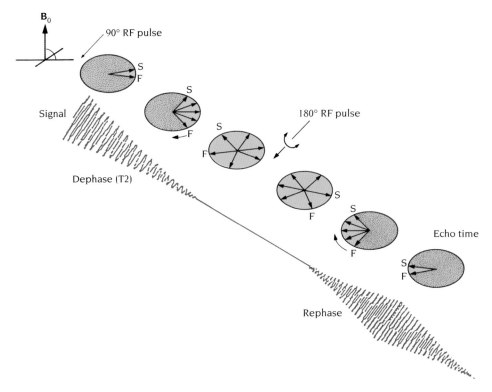

Figure 1-9. Spin-echo and T2 relaxation. After a 90° RF pulse, the protons are initially all directed along a single axis in the transverse plane and are said to be in phase. Thereafter, the faster-precessing and the slower-processing protons interact magnetically and their spins begin to dephase rapidly within the transverse plane so that their vectors spread to occupy an ever-enlarging sector and ultimately a disc. (What is illustrated is a pure T2 effect; the actual process involves a combination of T2 and T1 relaxation so that the disc illustrated becomes conical, as shown in Figure 1-10.) The application of a 180° refocusing pulse eliminates the effects of static magnetic field inhomogeneities, so that most spins are in phase at the first-echo time. Some residual dephasing is present at the echo owing to T2 effects, which cannot be reversed by the refocusing pulse. The 180° refocusing pulse can be repeated after the first echo is received (compare Figure 1-15). F, proton spins with faster precession; S, proton spins with slower precession. (Redrawn with permission from Edelman RR, Hesselink JR. Clinical Magnetic Resonance Imaging. Philadelphia, Pa: WB Saunders Co; 1990.)

of reference (Figure 1-9). The magnetic vectors thus spread out like the opening of a fan within the transverse plane from their initial location in one direction along the *y* axis. This process of loss of phase coherence among spins is called *transverse relaxation*. By convention, the transverse (spin-spin) relaxation time, or T2, is the time required for 63% of the magnetic field in the transverse plane created by the RF pulse to dissipate. This reflects the time-dependent interaction of proton spins, causing nuclei to precess at different rates and deviate from the uniform motion created on initial excitation.

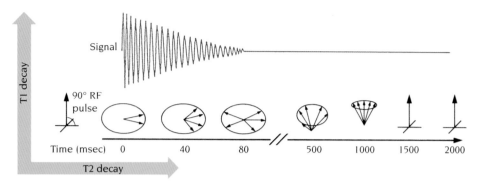

Figure 1-10. T1 and T2 relaxation compared. Following a single 90° RF pulse, T1 relaxation and T2 relaxation are simultaneous processes. Note that T2 relaxation is completed much more rapidly than T1 relaxation. The signal emitted represents both T1 and T2 relaxation according to the characteristics of the protons within the tissue. Note that the amplitude of the signal falls rapidly by the time the protons have dephased or are close to the transverse plane during T2 decay. (Redrawn with permission from Edelman RR, Hesselink JR. Clinical Magnetic Resonance Imaging. Philadelphia: WB Saunders Co; 1990.)

Longitudinal magnetization increases after the termination of the RF pulse (with a time constant of T1), while transverse magnetization decreases after the termination of the RF pulse (with a time constant of T2). T1 relaxation and T2 relaxation occur simultaneously, but T2 relaxation is completed much more rapidly than T1 relaxation (Figure 1-10). At the end of transverse relaxation, when the transverse magnetization has nearly reached zero, the magnetic vectors can be represented as located along the edge of a disc in the transverse plane. They are then brought into the shape of a cone of decreasing diameter during longitudinal relaxation. The tissue characteristics associated with T1 and T2 are discussed in Section 1-5.

1-4 TR AND TE DEFINED

An MRI examination protocol is described in part by the RF bursts used in its performance. The scanner operator performing the procedure sets the time between pulses, which is called the *repetition time* (TR). This represents the interval of time between cycles of excitation and relaxation. Allowing full longitudinal relaxation to occur (TR >> T1) after an RF pulse prolongs the examination time. However, repeating the RF pulse with TR less than the average T1 leads to reduced signal strength and a noisier image (Figure 1-11). These repeated patterns of RF bursts are called *pulse sequences*. Typical examples of pulse sequences used in MRI scanning are SR (saturation recovery), SE (spin-echo), and IR (inversion recovery).

Varying only TR affects the appearance of tissues. A series of 90° RF pulses followed by the immediate acquisition of the FID signal is shown in Figure 1-12. The illustration presumes that TR is much longer than T1, resulting in an equal FID amplitude after each pulse and thus indicating that complete relaxation occurred

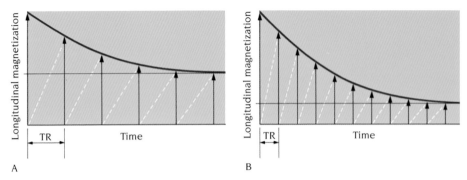

A   B

Figure 1-11. Equilibrium magnetization and magnetic saturation. (A) Greater equilibrium longitudinal magnetization results with a long TR between series of several RF pulses. (B) With a short TR, the equilibrium magnetization is less and the saturation of the protons is greater. In a series of repeated 90° pulses, a short TR is shown to decrease the residual or equilibrium amount of longitudinal magnetization, as compared to a long TR. Decreased equilibrium magnetization is associated with decreased signal strength on T1-weighted images. When 90° RF pulses are repeated with sufficiently rapid succession, the protons realign along the longitudinal meridian but without a net magnetic vector. When the protons align with equal numbers in the parallel and antiparallel directions, they are said to be saturated; this phenomenon forms the basis for saturation-recovery scanning. The *solid lines* represent the longitudinal relaxation following each pulse. *Top curve* (in color) connects the maximum relaxation at the end of each repetition.

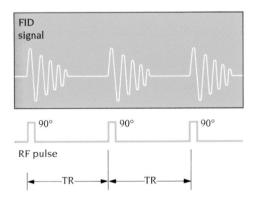

Figure 1-12. Signal produced by a train of RF pulses separated by a repetition time of TR. The free induction decay (FID) signal is measured immediately after each pulse.

prior to the next RF pulse. The signal intensity that is related to T1 relaxation time is illustrated in Figure 1-13, which has been calculated from data similar to those in Table 1-2. Note that the results can be considered in three regions: When TR < 2 sec, the relative signal intensities are white matter (WM) > gray matter (GM) and >> cerebrospinal fluid (CSF); when TR > 2 sec and < 5 sec, GM > WM > CSF; and when TR > 5 sec, CSF > GM > WM. The first pattern is T1-weighted and the last is described as proton-density-weighted.

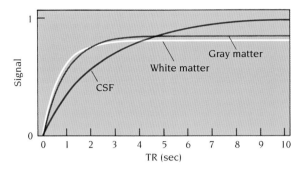

Figure 1-13. MRI signal calculated as a function of the pulse repetition time TR for gray matter (GM), white matter (WM), and cerebrospinal fluid (CSF), using the parameters of Table 1-1 and assuming typical relaxation times in proton densities. It is assumed that 90° pulses are applied every TRs and the signal is collected immediately thereafter. At short TR (TR < 2 sec), the relative signal intensities are WM > GM >> CSF and the resultant image is said to be T1-weighted. At longer TR (TR >2 sec and <5 sec), the relative signal intensities are GM > WM > CSF. Finally, at TR > 5 sec, the relative signal intensities are CSF > GM > WM and the resultant images are said to be proton-density-weighted. Gray matter and white matter are isointense when TR is approximately 2 sec and also below 0.5 sec. Note that CSF is essentially isointense with gray and white matter when TR is in the vicinity of 5 sec. If TR is allowed to become greater than 5 sec, CSF will have the highest signal intensity while the proton density of the gray and white matter will provide contrast for the brain. In this illustration, TE is held constant at 15 msec, causing CSF to have lower signal intensity than brain when TR < 5 sec. In clinical T2-weighted imaging, CSF has a higher signal than brain at TR > 2 sec because TE > 30 msec on second-echo images. Compare Figure 1-20. (Redrawn with permission from Atlas SW. Magnetic Resonance Imaging of the Brain and Spine. New York, NY: Raven Press; 1991.)

Saturation recovery (SR) sequences record the RF signal emitted by the protons after a series of 90° pulses with interpulse intervals approximately less than or equal to an average tissue T1, 0.1 to 1.5 sec (Figure 1-14). *Saturation* is defined in MRI as an equilibrium condition in which an equal number of protons are aligned with and against a magnetic field such that no further absorption of energy of the RF pulse will take place. Thus, the vector sum of all the proton magnetizations is zero and there is no net magnetic vector. Saturation can be produced by repeated pulses having interpulse intervals much shorter than T1. The effect of decreasing TR on the equilibrium magnetization series of pulses is shown in Figure 1-11. Repeating pulses more frequently than shown (i.e., reducing TR) will lead to saturation. Relaxation after the final pulse of such a series occurs from an initial condition of zero net magnetization, rather than from an initial condition of partial magnetization as would occur after a single RF pulse. Saturation-recovery techniques are used in T1-weighted scans of the sella to remove the effects of unsaturated protons in blood moving through the imaging volume. Saturation-recovery techniques also are useful in removing swallowing and respiratory motion artifacts.

Table 1-2. Factors Affecting MRI Signal Intensity

Protocol	Imaging Parameters			Relative Intensity of Signal					
	TI	TR	h	Bone/Air	Fat	Vitreous/CSF	Nerve/Muscle	Gray Matter	White Matter
Tl-weighted	None	600	15	0	++	--	+	-	+
T2-weighted	None	2500	90	0	--	+++	-	+	+
STIR	150	1500	20	0	--	++	++	++	
Proton density (%)					9.6	10.8	9.7	10.6	10.6

Top, Typical imaging parameters used in clinical magnetic resonance images of the orbit. Typical signal intensities for various tissues are compared. + Indicates brighter than average intensity; −, less than average intensity. *Bottom,* The proton densities of various tissues are shown and expressed as a percentage of MRI-visible protons in tissue compared with pure water. Note that the differences between tissues are small; this limits the usefulness of proton-density-weighted images.

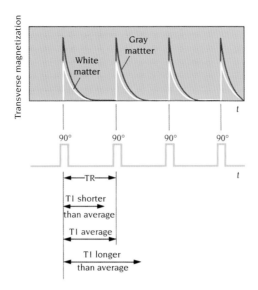

Figure 1-14. Saturation-recovery pulse sequence. A series of 90° RF pulses is given, separated by TR that is equal to average tissue T1. Relaxation is not complete between pulses. The tissue represented by the *curve printed in white* has a shorter T1 relaxation time than the tissue characterized by the *curve printed in gray*. Gray matter has a shorter T1 relaxation time than white matter. Because the FID signal will be related to the transverse magnetization, contrast on the printed image will result because the gray matter will produce a greater signal intensity than white matter for tissues of equal proton density.

SE (spin-echo) sequences use a similar set of pulses as SR sequences, with the addition of 180° pulses between the 90° pulses. SE techniques include an initial 90° pulse followed by one or more 180° pulses at equal intervals in succession, which generate first and subsequent echoes (or regenerations). The 180° pulse is given to alter the magnetization in the transverse plane, flipping the magnetic moment of the protons that have already been excited by the RF pulse while keeping them within the same plane. The resulting signal is sampled at a time TE (echo time) after the RF pulse, which is set by the operator to twice the interval between any two consecutive 180° pulses (see Figure 1-9).

The spin-echo technique minimizes the effects of inhomogeneities in the static magnetic field. The cycle can be thought of as flipping the protons into phase at the end of the pulse. The protons rapidly dephase due to the T2* relaxation but are brought back into phase (rephased) by the 180° RF pulse. The resultant signal is measured again. The T2 image is obtained in a later echo, on the order of 60 to 120 msec after the excitation (see Figure 1-15). First echo images (also called proton-density-weighted images) have also been commonly obtained in the past. However, these have mainly been replaced by FLAIR (fluid-attenuated inversion recovery) images except for specific indications that are outside the scope of this monograph.

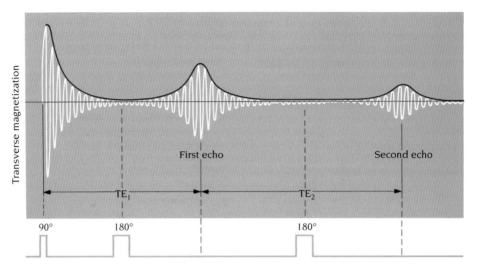

Figure 1-15. Use of a spin-echo technique to produce a T2-weighted signal due to signal decay (T2 contrast). The pulse sequence is a 90° RF pulse at the onset followed by two 180° RF refocusing pulses. The first 180° pulse is given at 1/2, the time at which the first echo will be recorded, and the second 180° pulse is given after the recording of the first signal and at half the time from the initial pulse to the time when the second echo will be recorded. The first and second echoes, TE_1 and TE_2, are asymmetric in this example.

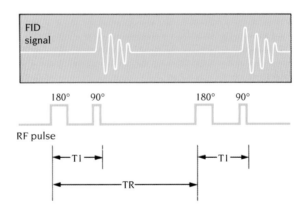

Figure 1-16. Inversion-recovery pulse sequence. The initial RF pulse is sufficient to provide a 180° inversion of the net magnetic vector of the protons and bring them into the nonequilibrium condition of antiparallel orientation. TI is the time interval between the inversion and the application of a 90° RF pulse. During TI, the proton spins relax partially, some of them returning to the parallel orientation. Because protons oriented in the longitudinal direction cannot be detected, they are flipped into the transverse plane by the application of the 90° pulse, where they produce a measurable signal.

Inversion recovery (IR) sequences use initial 180° pulses in the longitudinal plane prior to the standard 90° pulse and immediate acquisition of the FID signal (Figure 1-16). The time between the inversion and the 90° excitation is designated TI (not to be confused with the alphanumeric designation T1). TI is chosen such

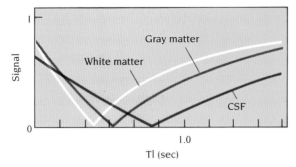

Figure 1-17. MRI signal calculated as a function of the inversion time TI, assuming a pulse TR of 2.5 sec and the parameters of Table 1-1 for gray matter, white matter, and cerebrospinal fluid (CSF). It is assumed that 90° pulses are applied every 2.5 sec and the signal is collected immediately after each pulse. Note the multiple crossover points at which gray matter, white matter, and CSF are predicted to be isointense. Furthermore, the inflection points at signal = 0 correspond to TI values, at which time the signal is nullified because the net magnetic vector is in the *x,y* plane halfway relaxed between the antiparallel and the parallel orientation. This occurs when TI = 0.69 TI of the tissue. (Redrawn with permission from Atlas SW. Magnetic Resonance Imaging of the Brain and Spine. New York, NY: Raven Press; 1991.)

that the longitudinal magnetization of a specific tissue is null. The latter cannot emit a signal (there is an absence of transverse magnetization due to the absence of longitudinal magnetization). The inversion-recovery technique thus allows the signal of a given tissue to be suppressed by selecting a TI adapted to the T1 of this tissue. Partial recovery of the longitudinal relaxation as a function of TR is measured in the transverse plane by the time of the application of the 90° RF pulse. In MRI examinations of the orbits, IR is often used with a short TI; this is designated a STIR (short tau inversion recovery) image. At an optimum TI (about 0.4 sec in Figure 1-17), white matter has very little signal. One of many fat-suppression techniques useful in imaging the orbit, STIR is especially valuable when combined with contrast agents, so that a contrast-enhanced tumor will produce an intense signal while normal bright orbital fat is suppressed on a T1-weighted image. A long IR is used to obtain FLAIR images, because water has a long T1, and this is especially valuable to review edematous lesions.

1-5 T1 AND T2 RELAXATION

Protons (hydrogen ions) are present in tissues as a consequence of the presence of water at tissue pH. Even without flow produced by external forces, free water molecules surrounding a hydrogen ion move rapidly and their rotational and translational Brownian movement produces rapid fluctuation in the magnetic fields adjacent to the protons. T2 relaxation times are fundamentally faster than T1 relaxation times. These molecular water–proton interactions accelerate T1 and T2 relaxation. Water molecules attached (bound) to proteins or to cell membranes (this is especially prominent in fat cells) move less rapidly than unattached (free) water molecules within tissue (Figure 1-18). Water molecules in flowing blood move rapidly. In adipose tissue and proteinaceous solutions, limited movement of water molecules occurs at a fluctuation rate equal to that of the resonant frequencies of the protons. Such solutions have rapid T1 and intermediate T2 relaxation times. However, in pure water, the molecules fluctuate more rapidly than the protons and do not affect them as much, giving pure water long T1 and T2 relaxation times, measured in seconds as opposed to milliseconds. When water molecules are very tightly bound to collagen in tendons and scar tissue, their slow fluctuation promotes rapid T2 relaxation but not T1 relaxation. Thus, such tissues have T2 relaxation times of less than 50 msec, while the T1 relaxation times may be in the vicinity of 1 sec. Slower-moving molecules, such as proteins, produce less rapid fluctuations in the magnetic field experienced by their protons and do not affect T1 relaxation as much as the faster-moving free water molecules. In biologic tissues, water is often bound to proteins, causing a change in the T1 relaxation of that protein. Efficient shortening of T1 relaxation occurs in the region of the curve representing the movement of water molecules bound to proteins and cell membranes, which restricts molecular motion compared to free water molecules. Perturbations in the bound-water and free-water content of tissues contribute to the contrast of abnormal from normal tissues.

I-6 FACTORS DETERMINING THE APPEARANCE OF MAGNETIC RESONANCE IMAGES

Image appearance of normal tissues on MRI depends on four major characteristics:

1. The proton density of structures contributes the majority of information concerning the structures. Tissues with higher proton density produce the most intense signals.
2. The time between the RF pulse and the sampling is represented in the parameters TR and TE and controls the T1 and T2 weighting of the images (Figure 1-19).
3. Flow is an important consideration in fluids that do not remain stationary. If protons are stimulated by the RF pulse and leave the slice being scanned before the image is sampled, then no signal will be obtained. Similarly, the protons that have come into the slice after the RF pulse have not been exposed to the pulse, and such protons will not contribute to the image. As a result, a flow void is seen where rapid flow exists. Thus, large vessels appear dark on typical T1- and T2-weighted images using spin-echo sequences unless special techniques are used to display them (i.e., MR angiography).
4. The electron clouds around atomic nuclei shield them from the applied magnetic field during the RF pulse, creating alterations in the local field that the nuclei encounter. For example, protons associated with water have a different Larmor frequency than protons associated with lipids because of differences in the electron cloud configuration.

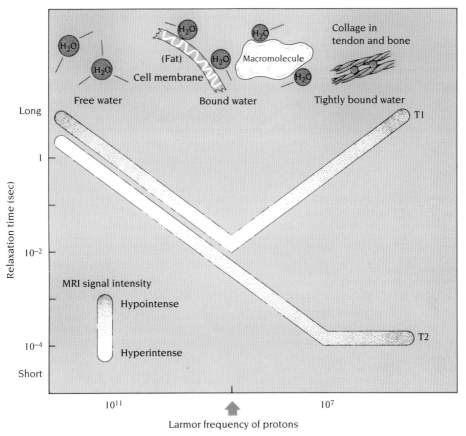

Figure 1-18. Relaxation time of protons versus frequency (Hz) of molecular motion of water molecules. Free water has rapid diffusion and long T1 and T2 times (free-water region). Bound water associated with restricted motion has shorter T1 and T2 times (bound-water region). Note that the T1 relaxation time of bound water is efficiently shortened as a function of its frequency of molecular motion. The clinical differentiation of biological fluids (cerebrospinal fluid and vitreous) from tissues occurs in the region represented by the right half of the bound-water region. Here T1 becomes much longer than T2. High signal intensity is represented by the light regions of the T1 and T2 curves. On T1-weighted images, high signal intensity is associated with short T1 times so that fatty tissue will be characteristically bright. On T2-weighted images, the high signal intensity is associated with long T2 times so that free water and edema in tissue will be characteristically bright. Note that free water molecules diffuse randomly in all directions. Bound water is associated with macromolecules and cell membranes and has T1 and T2 relaxation times that are shorter than those of free water. Collagen has tightly bound water with long T1 relaxation times and very short T2 relaxation times. (Redrawn and modified with permission from Edelman RR, Hesselink JR. Clinical Magnetic Resonance Imaging. Philadelphia, Pa: WB Saunders Co; 1990.)

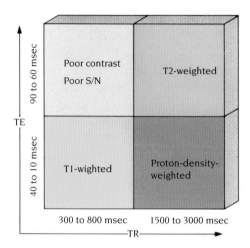

Figure 1-19. Image contrast as a function of TR and TE. *Bottom,* The 40- to 10-msec time corresponds to the first-echo times used clinically. *Top,* Corresponds to the second-echo times. *Right,* The TR shown corresponds to the TR used in a spin-echo technique, thus producing a proton-density-weighted scan on the first echo and a T2-weighted scan on the second echo. The T1-weighted signal is produced when TR is in the range shown on the *right.* S/N, signal-to-noise ratio. (Redrawn with permission from Edelman RR, Hesselink JR. Clinical Magnetic Resonance Imaging. Philadelphia: WB Saunders Co; 1990.)

Table 1-2 provides characteristics useful in differentiating the different types of MRI protocols. Note that gray matter and white matter have essentially equal proton densities, thus limiting the usefulness of this technique for differentiating normal anatomy. Look at the vitreous cavity and the CSF to make an initial evaluation of the weighting of a scan. If normal vitreous and CSF are hypointense, the scan is T1-weighted. The CSF can also be dark on a T2 FLAIR sequence because fluid signal is suppressed. If the CSF and vitreous are bright, then the scan is likely a T2-weighted study.

There is insufficient appreciation of the ability of MRI to adequately image bone and detect fractures. It is true that water molecules in cortical bone are tightly bound and few in number, producing no detectable signal. The black image of cortical bone can be appreciated as having contrast with regard to adjacent medullary bone, muscle, and fat. Moreover, hyperintense signals due to the intrusion of hemorrhage and edema into the normal low signal of cortical bone should alert to the presence of a fracture or tumor.

1-7 T1-WEIGHTED IMAGES

T1-weighted images (T1WI) are created by imaging with short TR values (200 to 1000 msec) and short TE values (15 to 25 msec). Because it is not feasible to use a TE of 0, all T1WIs have some degree of T2-weighting, which increases with a longer TE. Tissues that inherently have a shorter T1 will have greater signal intensity at a given TR than those with a longer T1 (Figure 1-20). Fat has a short T1, while gray matter, white matter, muscle, and CSF demonstrate increasingly long T1 relaxation times. T1-weighted images may provide better anatomic detail than T2-weighted images (T2WI) because the shorter time required to acquire images means less artifact induced by movement, including vascular pulsations of the brain.

T1 weighting is particularly good for imaging normal anatomic detail in the brain and orbit (Figures 1-21 to 1-56). Excellent contrast is observed between the high signal intensity of fat and the less intense signals of muscle and vessels. T1-weighted MRI can be useful for evaluating choroidal melanoma because the stable free radicals within melanin have paramagnetic properties that decrease both T1 and T2 relaxation times. This makes melanoma brighter on T1WI and darker on T2WI (Figure 1-57). The differential diagnosis for substances that are bright on the precontrast T1-weighted MR images includes proteinaceous fluid, fat, blood (depending on the stage), calcification, and melanin. The posterior pituitary gland can also demonstrate high signal on T1 (Figure 1-58).

The ophthalmologist cannot always rely on fat being bright on T1WI because special suppression sequences can suppress the normal hyperintense signal of fat on T1WI (i.e., "fat suppression," "fat saturation," or "water excitation") (Figures 1-59 to 1-68). The ophthalmologist must be familiar with these special scanning protocols to avoid misdiagnosis. The importance of this suppression sequence is

(*text continued on page 38*)

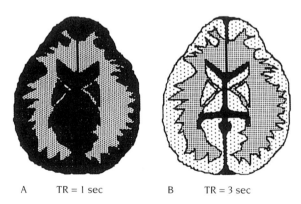

A   TR = 1 sec   B   TR = 3 sec

Figure 1-20. Theoretical MRI signal calculated as a function of the pulse repetition time (TR), assuming 90° pulses are applied every TR second and the signal is collected immediately thereafter. (A) T1-weighted (≈1 s). At short TR, the relative signal intensities are white matter (WM) > gray matter (GM) >> cerebrospinal fluid (CSF). The GM is relatively darker than the WM because it contains more water. (B) Proton-density-weighted (≈3 sec). At longer TR, the relative signal intensities are GM > WM > CSF. Note that GM and WM have reversed signal intensities but that the brain still has a higher signal than CSF. (Compare Figure 1-13, where TR = 1 sec corresponds to current A and TR = 3 sec corresponds to current B. Also compare Figure 1-21.) (Reprinted with permission from Latchaw RE. MR and CT Imaging of the Head, Neck and Spine. 2nd ed. St. Louis, Mo: Mosby–Year Book; 1991.)

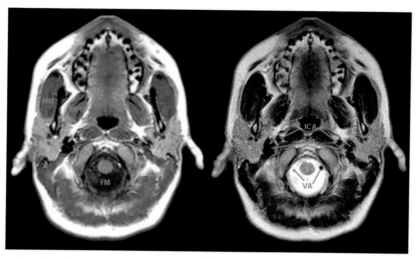

Figure 1-21. Axial T1-weighted (*left*) and T2-weighted (*right*) MRI of the cervical spinal cord just below the cervicomedullary junction demonstrating normal anatomy. Note the vertebral artery (VA) flow voids surrounded by bright cerebrospinal fluid signal on the T2-weighted study. FM, foramen magnum; ICA, internal carotid artery; IJV, internal jugular vein; MM, masseter muscle; MPM, medial pterygoid muscle; OcC, occipital condyle; SCo, spinal cord.

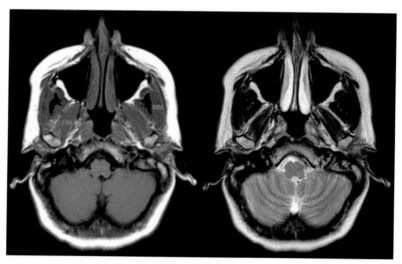

Figure 1-22. Axial T1-weighted (*left*) and T2-weighted (*right*) MRI of the normal medulla oblongata (MO) and cerebellar hemispheres (Cb). One common lesion in this location might be a lateral medullary infarct producing a Wallenberg syndrome clinically. LPM, lateral pterygoid muscle; MM, masseter muscle.

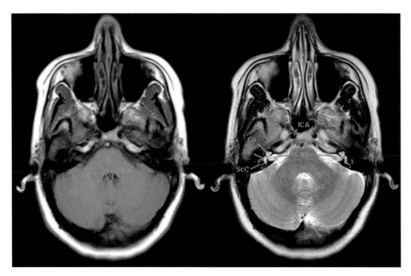

Figure 1-23. Axial T1-weighted (*left*) and T2-weighted (*right*) MRI demonstrating normal anatomy at the level of the pons (P). A lesion in the dorsal pons might produce a horizontal gaze palsy from involvement of the sixth cranial nerve nucleus, an internuclear ophthalmoplegia (INO) from a medial longitudinal fasciculus (MLF) lesion, or a "one-and-one-half" syndrome from involvement of both the sixth cranial nerve nuclei and the MLF. Note this is at the level of the sixth cranial nerve nucleus at the facial colliculus (FaC) visible bilaterally (formed by the seventh cranial nerve wrapping around the sixth cranial nerve nucleus). BA, basilar artery; C, clivus; Cb, cerebellum; CN8, eighth cranial nerve; Co, cochlea; ICA, internal carotid artery; MCP, middle cerebellar peduncle; ScC, semicircular canal; V4, fourth ventricle; Ve, vestibule.

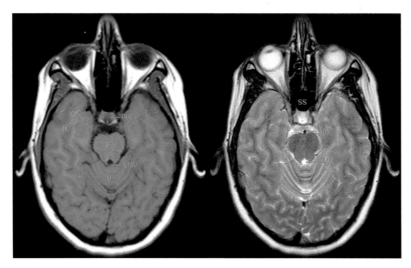

Figure 1-24. Axial T1-weighted (*left*) and T2-weighted (*right*) MRI demonstrating normal anatomy of the upper pons (P). Note how the vitreous and cerebrospinal fluid are dark on the T1-weighted image and bright on the T2-weighted image. BA, basilar artery; CaS, cavernous sinus; OL, occipital lobe; PiG, pituitary gland; SMV, superior medullary velum; SS, sphenoid sinus; TL, temporal lobe; V, vermis of cerebellum; V4, fourth ventricle.

27

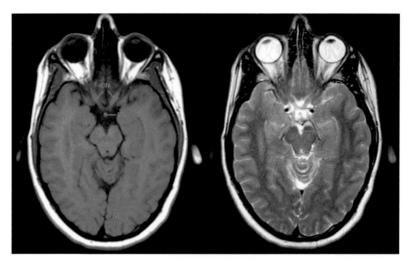

Figure 1-25. Axial T1-weighted (*left*) and T2-weighted (*right*) MRI demonstrating normal midbrain (MB) anatomy. A dorsal midbrain lesion might produce light near dissociation of the pupils, an upgaze paresis, and convergence-retraction nystagmus on attempted upgaze. The optic nerves (ON) can be seen approaching the optic chiasm (OC). The optic tracts (OT) are better visualized on the T2-weighted image when surrounded by bright cerebrospinal fluid (CSF) signal. Note the bright CSF signal also in the cerebral aqueduct (CA) on the T2-weighted image. ICi, interpeduncular cistern; OL, occipital lobe; PS, pituitary stalk; QCi, quadrigeminal cistern; TL, temporal lobe; U, uncus of temporal lobe; V, vermis of cerebellum.

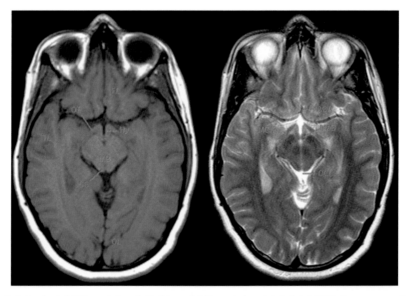

Figure 1-26. Axial T1-weighted (*left*) and T2-weighted (*right*) MRI demonstrating normal upper midbrain (MB) anatomy. The optic tract (OT), mamillary bodies (MaB), and superior colliculus (SC) can be seen on both the T1 and T2-weighted studies. The oculomotor nerve nucleus is located in the dorsal midbrain at the level of the superior colliculus. ACA, anterior cerebral artery; FL, frontal lobe; Hy, hypothalamus; MCA, middle cerebral artery; OL, occipital lobe; QCi, quadrigeminal cistern; TL, temporal lobe.

28

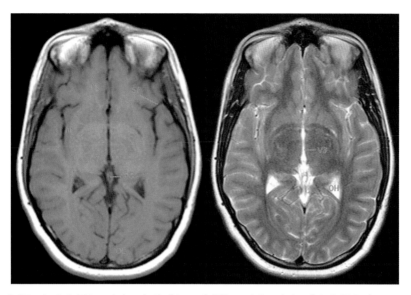

Figure 1-27. Axial T1-weighted (*left*) and T2-weighted (*right*) MRI demonstrating normal anatomy at the level of third ventricle (V3) between the two thalami (T). A thalamic lesion might produce a supranuclear vertical gaze palsy. FL, frontal lobe; In, insula; OH, occipital horn of lateral ventricle; OL, occipital lobe; PG, pineal gland; SF, sylvian fissure.

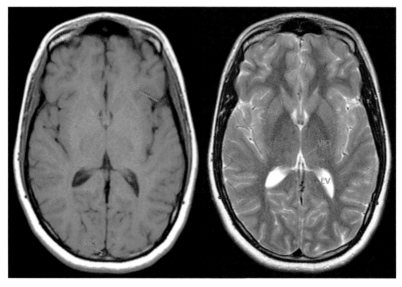

Figure 1-28. Axial T1-weighted (*left*) and T2-weighted (*right*) MRI demonstrating normal anatomy. The cistern of velum interpositum (VICi) is an anterosuperior extension of the quadrigeminal plate cistern. F, fornix; FL, frontal lobe; HCN, head of caudate nucleus; LV, lateral ventricle; OL, occipital lobe; Pu, putamen; SF, sylvian fissure; SSS, superior sagittal sinus.

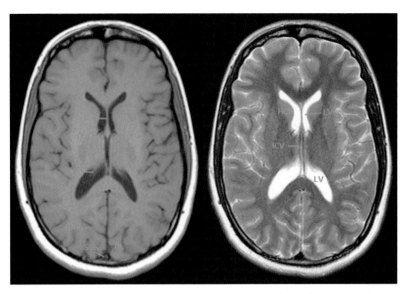

Figure 1-29. Axial T1-weighted *(left)* and T2-weighted *(right)* MRI demonstrating normal anatomy. Note the dark cerebrospinal fluid signal in the lateral ventricles on T1-weighted image and bright CSF signal on T2-weighted image. The genu (anterior) and splenium (posterior) of the corpus callosum (CC) are represented. The head of the caudate nucleus (HCN) indents the lateral aspect of the lateral ventricle (LV). The internal cerebral veins (ICV) are paired midline structures located in the roof of the third ventricle. ChP, choroid plexus; FL, frontal lobe; OL, occipital lobe; PoF, parieto-occipital fissure; SP, septum pellucidum; SSS, superior sagittal sinus.

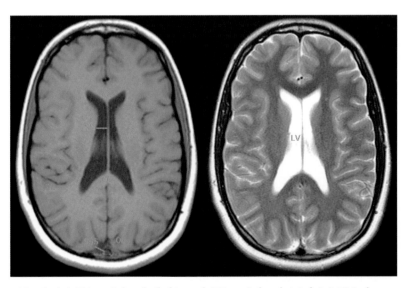

Figure 1-30. Axial T1-weighted *(left)* and T2-weighted *(right)* MRI demonstrating normal anatomy at the bodies of the lateral ventricle (LV). Note the septum pellucidum (SP), which may be absent in entities such as septo-optic dysplasia. CC, corpus callosum; CR, corona radiata; FL, frontal lobe; LV, lateral ventricle; OL, occipital lobe; PL, parietal lobe; SSS, superior sagittal sinus.

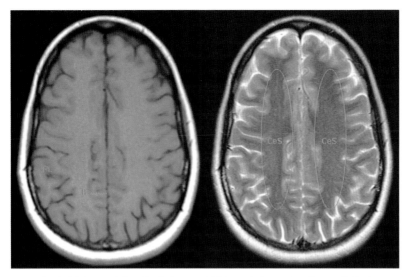

Figure 1-31. Axial T1-weighted (*left*) and T2-weighted (*right*) MRI demonstrating normal anatomy. White matter of the centrum semiovale (CeS) (*ovals*) can be affected by demyelinating lesions such as multiple sclerosis. FL, frontal lobe; IF, interhemispheric fissure; PL, parietal lobe.

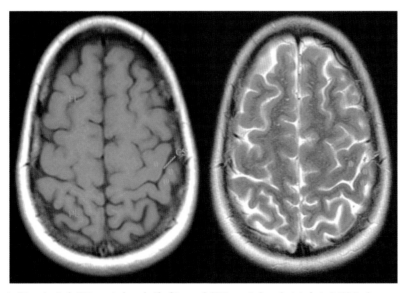

Figure 1-32. Axial T1-weighted (*left*) and T2-weighted (*right*) MRI demonstrating normal anatomy. The central sulcus (CS) separates the precentral motor cortex (*single dot*) from the postcentral sensory cortex (*double dots*). FL, frontal lobe; PL, parietal lobe.

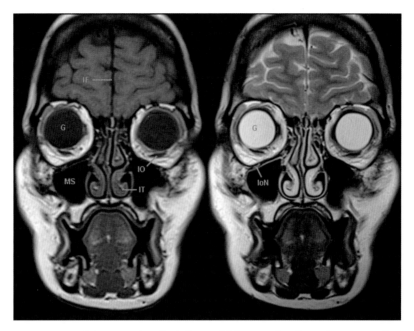

Figure 1-33. Coronal T1-weighted (*left*) and T2-weighted (*right*) MRI demonstrating normal mid-globe (G) anatomy. The inferior oblique muscle (IO) can be seen at this level. It arises from the medial aspect of the inferior orbital rim. Also seen is the infraorbital nerve (IoN) within the infraorbital canal in the floor of the orbit (*right*). G, globe; IF, interhemispheric fissure; IT, inferior turbinate; MS, maxillary sinus.

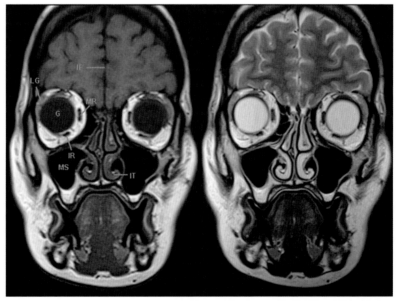

Figure 1-34. Coronal T1-weighted (*left*) and T2-weighted (*right*) MRI demonstrating normal anatomy also in the mid-globe (G) region (slightly posterior to Figure 1-33). Note the lacrimal gland (LG) evident in the superotemporal orbit. G, globe; IF, interhemispheric fissure; IR, inferior rectus muscle; IT, inferior turbinate; MR, medial rectus muscle; MS, maxillary sinus.

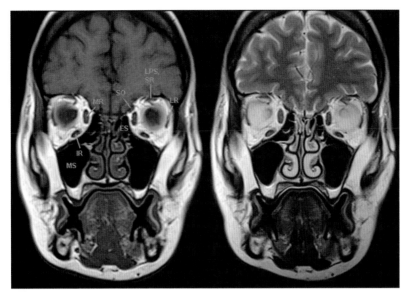

Figure 1-35. Coronal T1-weighted (*left*) and T2-weighted (*right*) MRI demonstrating normal anatomy at the level of the posterior globe. Note the various sizes of the extraocular muscles seen in cross section. ES, ethmoid sinus; IR, inferior rectus muscle; LPS, levator palpebrae superioris muscle; LR, lateral rectus muscle; MR, medial rectus muscle; MS, maxillary sinus; SO, superior oblique muscle; SR, superior rectus muscle.

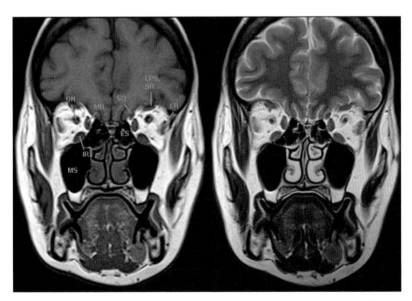

Figure 1-36. Coronal T1-weighted (*left*) and T2-weighted (*right*) MRI demonstrating normal orbital anatomy. Note the dark cerebrospinal fluid signal on the T1-weighted image immediately surrounding the normal optic nerve (ON) within the bright fat signal of the orbit. ES, ethmoid sinus; IR, inferior rectus muscle; LPS, levator palpebrae superioris muscle; LR, lateral rectus muscle; MR, medial rectus muscle; MS, maxillary sinus; SO, superior oblique muscle; SR, superior rectus muscle.

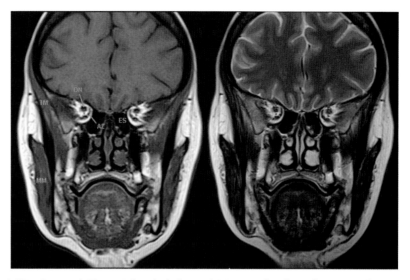

Figure 1-37. Coronal T1-weighted (*left*) and T2-weighted (*right*) MRI demonstrating normal anatomy at the orbital apex. Note the extraocular muscles form the annulus of Zinn (AZ) at this level. ES, ethmoid sinus; MM, masseter muscle; ON, optic nerve; TM, temporalis muscle.

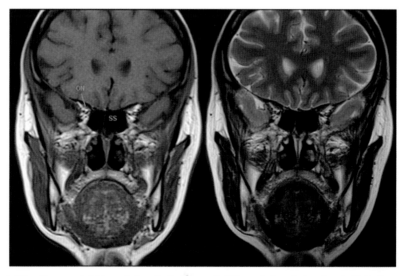

Figure 1-38. Coronal T1-weighted (*left*) and T2-weighted (*right*) MRI demonstrating normal posterior orbital apex anatomy. FH, frontal horn of lateral ventricle; ON, optic nerve; SS, sphenoid sinus.

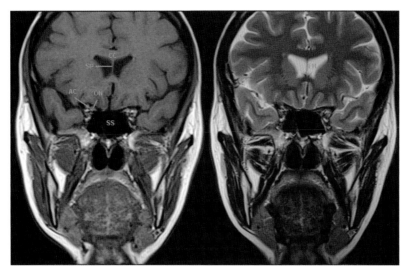

Figure 1-39. Coronal T1-weighted (*left*) and T2-weighted (*right*) MRI of the optic nerve (ON) within the optic canal demonstrating normal anatomy. AC, anterior clinoid process; CC, corpus callosum; FH, frontal horn of lateral ventricle; SP, septum pellucidum; SS, sphenoid sinus.

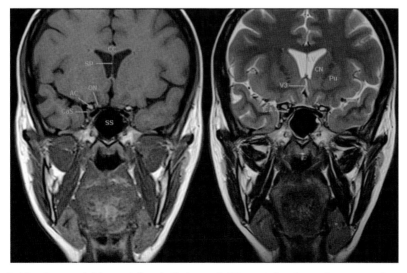

Figure 1-40. Coronal T1-weighted (*left*) and T2-weighted (*right*) MRI demonstrating normal intracranial optic nerve (ON) anatomy. Note the flow void (*black*) of the internal carotid artery (ICA) within the cavernous sinus (CaS). Also note the anterior clinoid process (AC), which is bright on T1-weighted imaging due to bone marrow fat within the process. CC, corpus callosum; CN, caudate nucleus; LV, lateral ventricle; Pu, putamen; SP, septum pellucidum; SS, sphenoid sinus; V3, third ventricle.

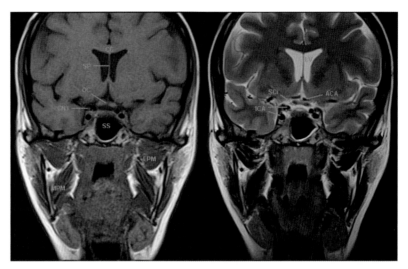

Figure 1-41. Coronal T1-weighted (*left*) and T2-weighted (*right*) MRI demonstrating normal anterior optic chiasm (OC) anatomy. Note the optic chiasm in the suprasellar cistern (SCi). ACA, anterior cerebral artery; CC, corpus callosum; CN3, third cranial nerve; ICA, internal carotid artery; LPM, lateral pterygoid muscle; LV, lateral ventricle; MPM, medial pterygoid muscle; SP, septum pellucidum; SS, sphenoid sinus.

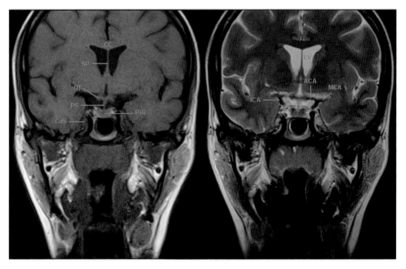

Figure 1-42. Coronal T1-weighted (*left*) and T2-weighted (*right*) MRI of the normal posterior optic chiasm. Note the supraclinoid internal carotid artery (ICA) just prior to its bifurcation. The pituitary stalk (PS) is also seen. The pituitary gland (PiG) is seen within the sella turcica and lies approximately 10 mm below the optic chiasm. Before visual field defects become apparent, pituitary lesions must be large enough to break through the diaphragma sellae and extend into the suprasellar cistern, where they compress the visual pathway commonly producing bitemporal hemianopic field defects. ACA, anterior cerebral artery; CaS, cavernous sinus; CC, corpus callosum; ICA, internal carotid artery; LV, lateral ventricle; MCA, middle cerebral artery; OT, optic tract; SP, septum pellucidum.

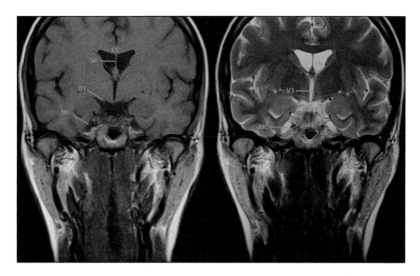

Figure 1-43. Coronal T1-weighted (*left*) and T2-weighted (*right*) MRI at the level of the third ventricle (V3) demonstrating normal anatomy. Cerebrospinal fluid within the Meckel caves (MC) is visualized bilaterally (dark on T1- and bright on T2-weighted imaging). CC, corpus callosum; LV, lateral ventricle; OT, optic tract; SP, septum pellucidum.

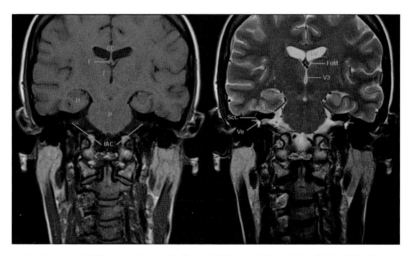

Figure 1-44. Coronal T1-weighted (*left*) and T2-weighted (*right*) MRI demonstrating normal anatomy. Note several structures of the inner ear at this level, the semicircular canal (ScC) and vestibule (Ve), seen best on the T2-weighted image. ACi, ambient cistern; CC, corpus callosum; F, fornix; FoM, foramen of Monro; H, hippocampus; IAC, internal auditory canal; LV, lateral ventricle; P, pons; T, thalamus; V3, third ventricle; VA, vertebral artery.

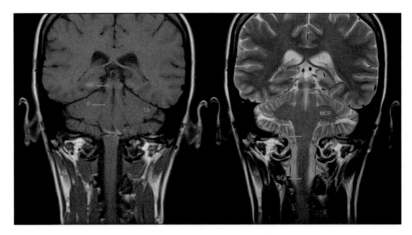

Figure 1-45. Coronal T1-weighted (*left*) and T2-weighted (*right*) MRI demonstrating normal anatomy at the level of the middle cerebellar peduncle (MCP). CA, cerebral aqueduct; Cb, cerebellum; ICV, internal cerebral vein; LV, lateral ventricle; MB, midbrain; MO, medulla oblongata; P, pons; SCo, spinal cord.

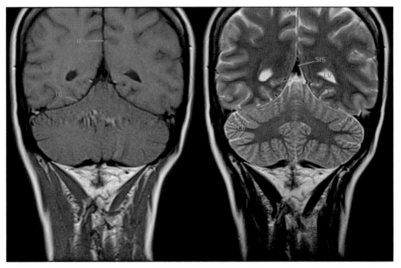

Figure 1-46. Coronal T1-weighted (*left*) and T2-weighted (*right*) MRI demonstrating normal anatomy of the cerebellum (Cb). The tentorium cerebelli (TC) is a crescentic, arched, duplicated dural membrane that covers the cerebellum and supports the occipital lobe. IF, interhemispheric fissure; LV, lateral ventricle; StS, straight sinus; V, vermis of cerebellum.

to eliminate or reduce the bright signal from normal tissue in order to enhance visualization of underlying pathology that might be obscured by the hyperintense signal of fat. Fat suppression sequences allow better visualization of underlying pathologic lesions on T1WI of the orbit, particularly after contrast has been administered. Without fat suppression, the overlying bright fat T1 signal might obscure underlying contrast enhancement (e.g., optic nerve enhancement in optic

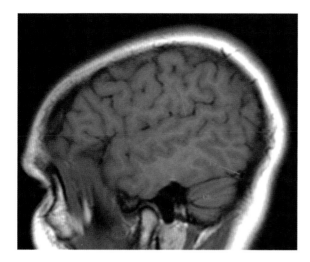

Figure 1-47. Parasagittal T1-weighted MRI demonstrating normal anatomy. Cb, cerebellum; SF, sylvian fissure; TL, temporal lobe; TS, transverse sinus.

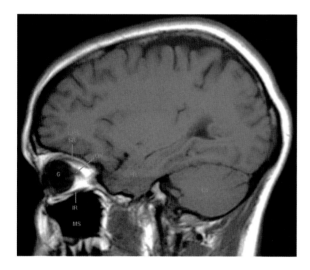

Figure 1-48. Parasagittal T1-weighted MRI demonstrating normal orbital anatomy. Cb, cerebellum; G, globe; IR, inferior rectus muscle; LPS, levator palpebrae superioris muscle; MS, maxillary sinus; ON, optic nerve; SR, superior rectus muscle; TL, temporal lobe.

neuritis or optic nerve sheath meningioma) (Figure 1-69). Fat suppression techniques can also confirm the content of fat-containing lesions, such as dermoid cysts (Figure 1-70) and lipomas. Although the ophthalmologist does not have to order T1 fat-suppressed images, they should strongly consider fat suppression for all postcontrast orbital MR scans (e.g., for evaluation of optic nerve sheath meningioma or optic neuritis). At most centers, postcontrast imaging with fat suppression is an established protocol. Ophthalmologists should be aware that inadequate or incomplete fat suppression can be caused by metallic artifact (e.g., braces, metal in mascara) and at the air–bone interface of adjacent paranasal

(*text continued on page 42*)

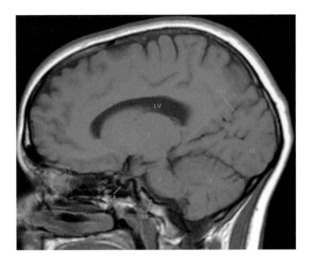

Figure 1-49. Parasagittal T1-weighted MRI demonstrating normal anatomy. Note the S-shaped course of the internal carotid artery (ICA), which marks the location of the cavernous sinus. Also note the basilar artery (BA) flow void (*black*). Cb, cerebellum; CC, corpus callosum; LV, lateral ventricle; OL, occipital lobe; P, pons; PoF, parieto-occipital fissure; T, thalamus.

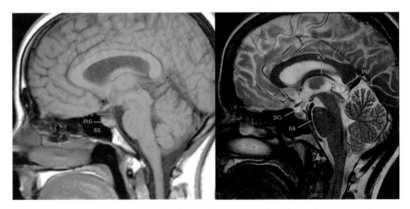

Figure 1-50. Sagittal T1-weighted (*left*) and T2-weighted (*right*) MRI demonstrating normal anatomy. Increased T2 signal is demonstrated within the pineal gland consistent with a pineal cyst. BA, basilar artery; C, clivus; CA, cerebral aqueduct; Cb, cerebellum; CC, corpus callosum; CT, cerebellar tonsil; IC, inferior colliculus; ICV, internal cerebral vein; LV, lateral ventricle; MaB, mamillary body; MB, midbrain; MO, medulla oblongata; OC, optic chiasm; P, pons; PG, pineal gland; PiG, pituitary gland; PS, pituitary stalk; QCi, quadrigeminal cistern; SC, superior colliculus; SCi, suprasellar cistern; SCo, spinal cord; SMV, superior medullary velum; SS, sphenoid sinus; T, thalamus; V3, third ventricle; V4, fourth ventricle.

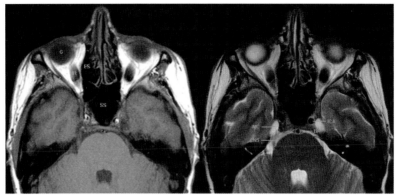

Figure 1-51. Axial T1-weighted (*left*) and T2-weighted (*right*) MRI demonstrating normal anatomy of inferior orbit. It may be difficult to differentiate the inferior orbit from the superior orbit without identifying adjacent structures such as the paranasal sinuses. BA, basilar artery; CN5, fifth cranial nerve; ES, ethmoid sinus; G, globe; ICA, internal carotid artery; IR, inferior rectus muscle; LR, lateral rectus muscle; MC, Meckel cave.

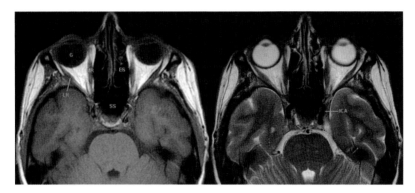

Figure 1-52. Axial T1-weighted (*left*) and T2-weighted (*right*) MRI of the normal orbit at a level just inferior to the optic nerve. BA, basilar artery; ES, ethmoid sinus; G, globe; ICA, internal carotid artery; LR, lateral rectus muscle; MR, medial rectus muscle; SS, sphenoid sinus.

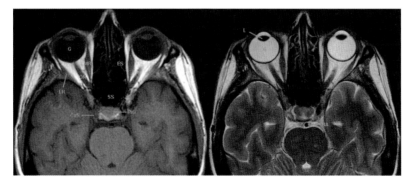

Figure 1-53. Axial T1-weighted (*left*) and T2-weighted (*right*) MRI demonstrating normal mid-orbit anatomy. BA, basilar artery; CaS, cavernous sinus; ES, ethmoid sinus; G, globe; L, lens; LR, lateral rectus muscle; MR, medial rectus muscle; ON, optic nerve; PiG, pituitary gland; SS, sphenoid sinus.

41

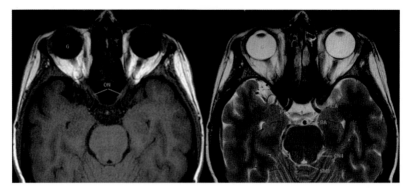

Figure 1-54. Axial T1-weighted (*left*) and T2-weighted (*right*) MRI demonstrating normal orbital anatomy. Note the course of the optic nerve (ON) through the optic canal. The fourth cranial nerve (CN4) decussates and exits the brainstem dorsally in the region of the superior medullary velum (SMV), beneath the inferior colliculus. Traumatic fourth cranial nerve palsies have been attributed to injury in the area of the posterior decussation from contact with the edge of the tentorium cerebelli. BA, basilar artery; G, globe; ICA, internal carotid artery; MR, medial rectus muscle; PS, pituitary stalk.

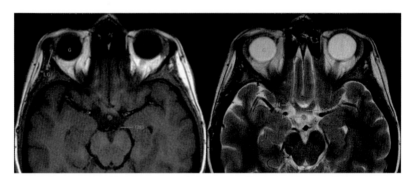

Figure 1-55. Axial T1-weighted (*left*) and T2-weighted (*right*) MRI demonstrating normal anatomy of the superior orbit. Note the optic chiasm (OC) and adjacent structures. CN3, third cranial nerve; G, globe; LG, lacrimal gland; ON, optic nerve; PS, pituitary stalk.

sinuses due to the magnetic field changes at air–tissue interfaces (i.e., high signal area at the inferior rectus muscle adjacent to very low signal air in the maxillary sinus). This hyperintense signal artifact could be misinterpreted as abnormal enhancement and the ophthalmologist should be suspicious of reports of orbital MR describing "abnormal enhancement" in this area (e.g., "orbital inflammatory pseudotumor" or "orbital enhancement in inferior rectus muscle"), especially if there is no clinical correlate and there is visible metallic artifact on the ipsilateral side. Careful review of other sequences might confirm that the abnormal signal is indeed artifact.[32–35]

(*text continued on page 49*)

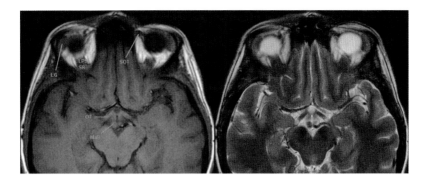

Figure 1-56. Axial T1-weighted (*left*) and T2-weighted (*right*) MRI demonstrating normal anatomy of the superior orbit. LG, lacrimal gland; LPS, levator palpebrae superioris muscle; MaB, mamillary body; OT, optic tract; SOT, superior oblique muscle tendon; SR, superior rectus muscle.

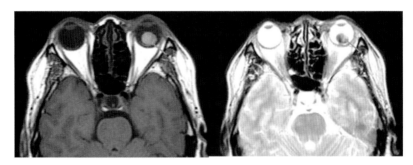

Figure 1-57. Axial T1-weighted (*left*) and T2-weighted (*right*) MRI demonstrating a choroidal melanoma (*arrows*). Note the melanoma is bright on unenhanced T1-weighted imaging and dark on T2-weighted imaging consistent with its melanin content.

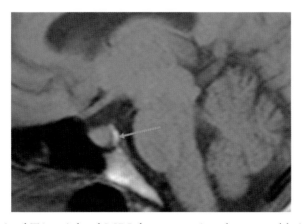

Figure 1-58. Sagittal T1-weighted MRI demonstrating the normal bright signal of the posterior pituitary gland (*arrow*).

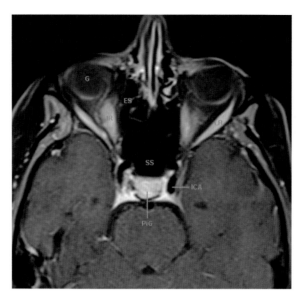

Figure 1-59. Axial postcontrast T1-weighted MRI with fat suppression demonstrating normal anatomy of the inferior orbit. ES, ethmoid sinus; G, globe; ICA, internal carotid artery; IR, inferior rectus muscle; LR, lateral rectus muscle; PiG, pituitary gland; SS, sphenoid sinus.

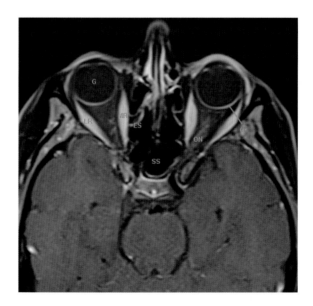

Figure 1-60. Axial postcontrast T1-weighted MRI with fat suppression demonstrating normal anatomy of the mid-orbit. Note the loss of the usual bright fat signal in the orbit and subcutaneous tissue with this fat suppression sequence (compare Figure 1-53, left). Also note enhancement of the highly vascular extraocular muscles and choroid (Ch). ES, ethmoid sinus; G, globe; LR, lateral rectus muscle; MR, medial rectus muscle; ON, optic nerve; SS, sphenoid sinus.

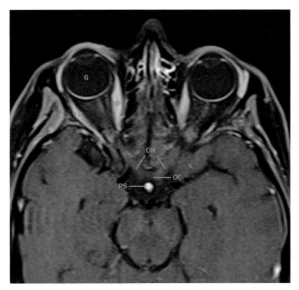

Figure 1-61. Axial postcontrast T1-weighted MRI with fat suppression demonstrating normal orbital anatomy at the level of the optic chiasm (OC). G, globe; LR, lateral rectus muscle; MR, medial rectus muscle; ON, optic nerve; PS, pituitary stalk.

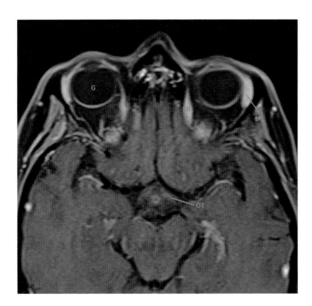

Figure 1-62. Axial postcontrast T1-weighted MRI with fat suppression demonstrating normal anatomy of the superior orbit. G, globe; LG, lacrimal gland; MR, medial rectus muscle; OT, optic tract.

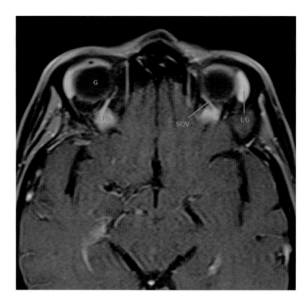

Figure 1-63. Axial postcontrast T1-weighted MRI with fat suppression demonstrating normal anatomy of the superior orbit. G, globe; LG, lacrimal gland; LPS, levator palpebrae superioris muscle; SOV, superior ophthalmic vein; SR, superior rectus muscle.

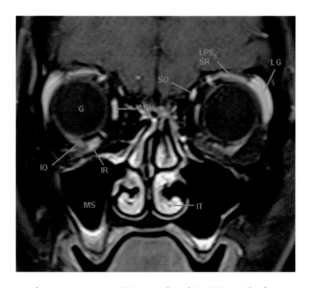

Figure 1-64. Coronal postcontrast T1-weighted MRI with fat suppression demonstrating normal mid-globe anatomy. G, globe; IO, inferior oblique muscle; IR, inferior rectus muscle; IT, inferior turbinate; LG, lacrimal gland; LPS, levator palpebrae superioris muscle; MR, medial rectus muscle; MS, maxillary sinus; SO, superior oblique muscle; SR, superior rectus muscle.

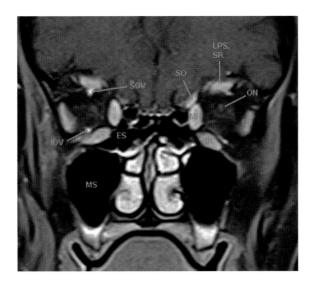

Figure 1-65. Coronal postcontrast T1-weighted MRI with fat suppression demonstrating normal orbital anatomy. ES, ethmoid sinus; IOV, inferior ophthalmic vein; IR, inferior rectus muscle; LPS, levator palpebrae superioris muscle; LR, lateral rectus muscle; MS, maxillary sinus; ON, optic nerve; SO, superior oblique muscle; SOV, superior ophthalmic vein; SR, superior rectus muscle.

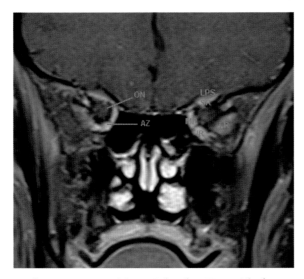

Figure 1-66. Coronal postcontrast T1-weighted MRI with fat suppression demonstrating normal orbital apex anatomy. AZ, annulus of Zinn; IR, inferior rectus muscle; LPS, levator palpebrae superioris muscle; LR, lateral rectus muscle; MR, medial rectus muscle; ON, optic nerve; SR, superior rectus muscle.

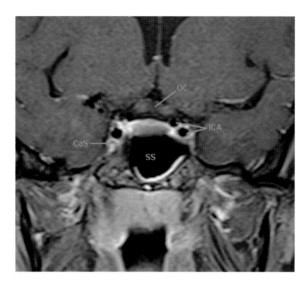

Figure 1-67. Coronal postcontrast T1-weighted MRI with fat suppression demonstrating normal anatomy at the level of the anterior optic chiasm (OC). CaS, cavernous sinus; ICA, internal carotid artery; OC, optic chiasm; SS, sphenoid sinus.

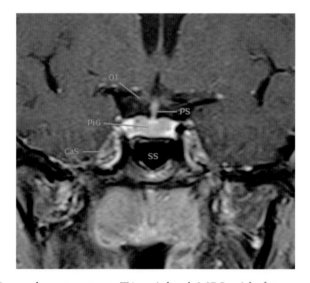

Figure 1-68. Coronal postcontrast T1-weighted MRI with fat suppression demonstrating normal anatomy at the level of the posterior optic chiasm. CaS, cavernous sinus; OT, optic tract; PiG, pituitary gland; PS, pituitary stalk; SS, sphenoid sinus.

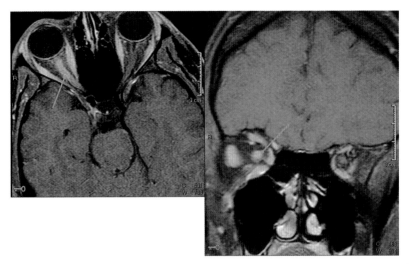

Figure 1-69. Axial (*left*) and coronal (*right*) postcontrast T1-weighted MRI with fat suppression demonstrating optic nerve enhancement (*arrows*) in a patient with acute optic neuritis. Without fat suppression, optic nerve enhancement may not be appreciated as it could be obscured by the surrounding bright orbital fat signal on T1-weighted imaging.

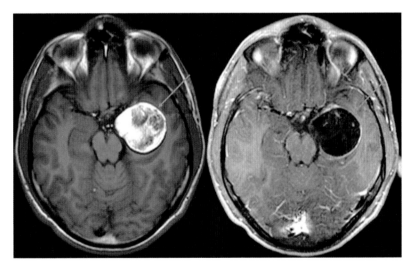

Figure 1-70. Axial precontrast, non–fat-suppressed T1-weighted MRI (*left*) demonstrating bright, heterogeneous signal in a left temporal lobe dermoid cyst. With fat suppression, the lesion loses its bright signal on the axial postcontrast T1-weighted MRI (*right*), indicative of its fat content.

1-8 T2-WEIGHTED IMAGES

Increasing TR to greater than 2000 msec and the second TE to greater than 70 msec produces an image with T2-weighting. Because TR is set at a value much greater than an average T1, most of the T1 effect is eliminated. However, eliminating T1 characteristics altogether would increase scanning time considerably. As a result, T2WI still possesses some minimal T1 characteristics. Tissues with low T2 values lose their signal more rapidly than do those with high T2 values, because T2 is a measure of the dephasing of the proton spins (see Figures 1-15 and 1-71). The rapidly dephasing protons in tissues with short T2 times emit a wide range of frequencies that are excluded by the receiver, which is narrowly tuned to the Larmor frequency. As a result, the long T2 tissues have a brighter signal than that of the short T2 tissues—the opposite of T1. To express it another way, those tissues whose protons slowly dephase have a long T2 and a high intensity signal. Examples include water and CSF. T2WI are less useful for fine anatomic detail than T1WI because of the increased time required for acquisition (see Figures 1-21 to 1-46 and 1-50 to 1-56). However, because of the hyperintense signal associated with perturbations of free water and bound water in tissues affected by edema, demyelination, and tumor infiltration, T2WI are frequently used to screen the brain for disease, demonstrating these changes more dramatically than T1 weighting (see Figure 1-18).

T2-weighted pathologic lesions include demyelinating pathology (e.g., periventricular white matter lesions in multiple sclerosis), ischemia (e.g., stroke), inflammatory disease, toxic or metabolic disorders (e.g., Wernicke encephalopathy), and neoplasms. Due to the CSF signal being bright on T2WI, certain lesions that are adjacent to CSF spaces are better seen when there is suppression of the CSF signal. This is done with the FLAIR sequence and improves visualization of subtle adjacent or underlying pathologic hyperintensity on T2WI (e.g., periventricular white matter demyelination or posterior reversible encephalopathy). Like fat-suppression sequences in T1WI, the ophthalmologist should not mistake a FLAIR study for a T1WI just because the CSF appears dark, as FLAIR is designed to suppress the normal CSF signal. It is unlikely that an ophthalmologist would have to specifically order FLAIR as most radiology facilities routinely perform this sequence as part of a standard protocol in MRI.

1-9 COMPUTED TOMOGRAPHY VERSUS MAGNETIC RESONANCE IMAGING OF HEMORRHAGE

CT is generally the best way to detect acute hemorrhage, especially when it is located in the cerebral ventricles or the subarachnoid space (Figure 1-72). Acute hemorrhage (less than 6 hr in duration) usually appears bright on noncontrast CT due to attenuation of the x-rays by hemoglobin. Subacute intraparenchymal blood is often isodense with brain on CT scans. In the chronic stage following bleeding (more than 2 weeks), intraparenchymal changes and loss of tissue cause the affected area to appear dark. The progression of intraparenchymal hemorrhage on MRI scanning is compared with that on CT in Table 1-3. Note that by the time of the subacute stage (approximately 1 week), MRI becomes the preferred method of examination for hemorrhage.

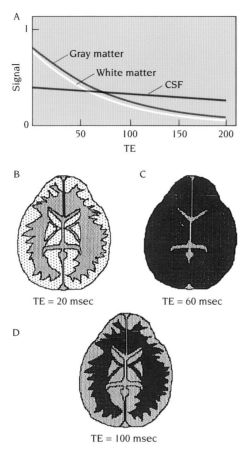

Figure 1-71. The signal intensity on T2-weighted scans is a function of echo time for the spin-echo pulse sequence. (A) Theoretical brain signal versus echo time (msec, TE) calculated on the basis of TR = 2 sec. The high signal intensity results from the narrow frequency spectrum emitted by the protons precessing in phase that result in a long T2 signal. The rapidly dephasing protons in tissues with short T2 times emit a wide range of frequencies that are excluded by the receiver, which is narrowly tuned to the Larmor frequency. Note that the cerebrospinal fluid (CSF) will be relatively bright at longer echo times only because fat, gray matter, white matter, muscle, and tightly bound water in tissue all dephase even more quickly. At shorter echo times, CSF has a lower signal intensity due to its long T1. However, as TE increases, the CSF signal intensity eventually surpasses that of gray and white matter (GM and WM, respectively) due to its very long T2 (approximately 1500 msec versus 80 and 70 msec for GM and WM, respectively). The brain contrasts shown in B, C, and D correspond to TEs of approximately 20 msec (GM > WM >> CSF), 60 msec (GM = CSF > WM), and 100 msec (CSF > GM > WM). This last image is said to be T2-weighted. (Reprinted with permission from Latchaw RE. MR and CT Imaging of the Head, Neck and Spine. 2nd ed. St. Louis, Mo: Mosby–Year Book; 1991.)

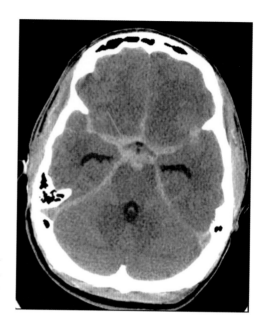

Figure 1-72. Axial noncontrast CT scan demonstrating diffuse subarachnoid space hyperdensity consistent with acute subarachnoid hemorrhage (*arrow*).

Table 1-3 MRI and CT Appearance in the Center of an Intraparenchymal Cerebral Hemorrhage

Time (Variable)	Biochemical/Cellular Basis	MRI Intensity		CT Density
		T1-Weighted	T2-Weighted	
Active	Intracellular Fe^{++} oxyhemoglobin	Isodense/ Hypodense	Isodense/ Hypodense	Bright/ isodense
Hyperacute	Intracellular Fe^{++} oxyhemoglobin	Isodense/ Hypodense	Hyperdense	Bright
	Deoxyhemoglobin	Isodense/ Hypodense	Hypodense	
Acute	Intracellular Fe^{++} deoxyhemoglobin	Isodense	Hypodense	Bright
Late acute	Intracellular Fe^{++} methemoglobin	Hyperdense	Hypodense	Bright/ isodense
Subacute	Extracellular Fe^{+++} methemoglobin after cell lysis	Hyperdense	Hyperdense	Isodense
Chronic	Methemoglobin (center)	Hyperdense	Hyperdense	Dark/ isodense
	Hemosiderin (periphery)	Isodense	Hypodense	

Although CT is considered superior to MRI for demonstrating acute hemorrhage, special MR sequences, such as gradient echo (GRE), can also show acute blood products effectively. GRE sequences are performed without the rephasing pulse, which causes susceptibility to inhomogeneities, such as blood. Even trace amounts of hemorrhage may be detected due to the profound signal loss caused by

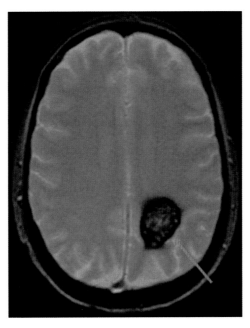

Figure 1-73. Gradient echo MRI demonstrating a hypointense mass consistent with hemorrhage in a left occipital cavernous malformation. Even trace amounts of hemorrhage may be detected due to the profound signal loss caused by the paramagnetic effects of deoxyhemoglobin and methemoglobin.

the paramagnetic effects of deoxyhemoglobin and methemoglobin. By using GRE, along with T1WI and T2WI, the approximate age of a hematoma may be determined.[1] GRE MR sequences might be useful to demonstrate hemorrhage in cases of arteriovenous or cavernous malformation (Figure 1-73), intracerebral hemorrhage, or traumatic brain injury. Evolving GRE imaging techniques, in combination with FLAIR and T2WI, have shown promise in detecting subarachnoid hemorrhage. CT also does not give as much information as MRI concerning the location of subacute blood or the presence of an underlying lesion producing the hemorrhage (e.g., arteriovenous malformation, aneurysm, stroke, or tumor). MRI can also detect small hemorrhages, especially those in the posterior fossa that could be missed by CT due to bone artifact. Moreover, MR angiography is readily combined to give additional information concerning abnormal vessel configurations and thrombosed veins.

1-10 DIFFUSION-WEIGHTED IMAGING

Diffusion-weighted imaging (DWI) is a special MRI technique that is based on the microscopic random Brownian motion of water. These changes in water molecular diffusion can be measured as signal intensity in vivo with DWI. In certain pathologic states, diffusion becomes restricted (hyperintense or "bright" on

DWI). The mobility of water within intracranial tissue is called the *apparent diffusion coefficient* (ADC). The combination of DWI and ADC can define specific pathology of water diffusion. Thus, DWI can differentiate the various phases of cerebral infarction: hyperacute, acute, subacute, and chronic. In the hyperacute phase, there is restricted diffusion (hyperintense on DWI) and decreased ADC, often with normal T2WI and FLAIR sequences. During the acute phase, there is also restricted diffusion and decreased ADC, but there is typically hyperintensity on T2WI (Figure 1-74). In the subacute phase, DWI may still be bright but ADC values are normal. Finally, in the chronic phase, the DWI shows hypointensity and the ADC is increased. Thus, DWI can detect hyperacute ischemic stroke even before abnormalities are detected on conventional T1- and T2-weighted MR sequences.

For the ordering ophthalmologist, the most common applications for using DWI/ADC are acute ischemic homonymous hemianopsia, cortical visual impairment, evidence of acute cerebral emboli in a patient with embolic retinal arterial occlusion, and top of the basilar syndrome with acute brainstem ischemia producing a progressive ophthalmoplegia. DWI/ADC can discriminate reversible vasogenic from irreversible cytotoxic edema. In vasogenic edema, the diffusion of water molecules is increased, so the ADC is elevated and the DWI shows isointense or hypointense signal. In contrast, in cytotoxic edema the movement of water from the extracellular to the intracellular compartment produces restricted diffusion, so the ADC is decreased and the DWI appears hyperintense. The scenario in which the ophthalmologist might be faced with the question of vasogenic versus cytotoxic edema is in posterior reversible encephalopathy syndrome (PRES) (Figure 1-75). PRES produces

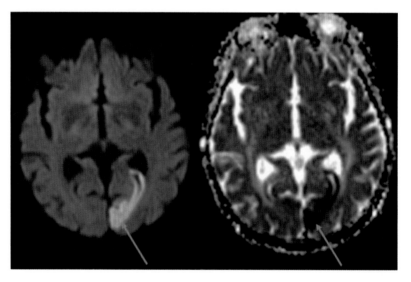

Figure 1-74. Diffusion weighted imaging (*left*) demonstrating an area of bright signal, which is dark on the corresponding apparent diffusion coefficient map (*right*), consistent with a hyperacute cerebral infarct of the left occipital cortex.

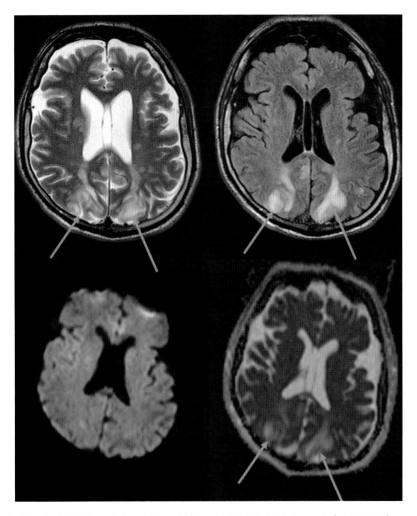

Figure 1-75. Axial T2-weighted (*top left*) and T2 FLAIR (*top right*) MRI demonstrating bilateral, symmetric posterior occipital lobe hyperintensities (*arrows*), which are not bright on diffusion-weighted imaging (*bottom left*) but are bright on apparent diffusion coefficient map (*bottom right; arrows*), consistent with vasogenic rather than cytotoxic edema in posterior reversible encephalopathy syndrome (PRES).

vasogenic edema that typically affects the posterior brain (e.g., occipital lobes) and can result in a homonymous hemianopsia or cortical visual impairment. Posterior reversible encephalopathy syndrome is usually seen in the setting of hypertension or eclampsia, but immunosuppressive medications (e.g., cyclosporine and tacrolimus) can produce a similar radiographic picture. Other DWI/ADC applications include assessment of inflammatory (e.g., brain abscess and vasculitis), degenerative (e.g., Alzheimer dementia), demyelinating (e.g., multiple sclerosis), and neoplastic lesions (e.g., differentiating epidermoid versus arachnoid cyst).[2–7]

1-11 PERFUSION-WEIGHTED IMAGING

Perfusion-weighted imaging (PWI) provides additional information about stroke pathophysiology and is useful in decision making for using interventional therapy in acute ischemic strokes (e.g., thrombolytic therapy).[2-9] PWI allows measurement of capillary perfusion in an area of interest by signal tracking after the bolus injection of a paramagnetic contrast agent and requires ultrafast MR sequences.[10] PWI provides information about cerebrovascular hemodynamic parameters, such as cerebral blood volume (CBV), time to peak (TTP), mean transit time (MTT), and cerebral blood flow (CBF)[1] (Figure 1-76). The volume difference of DWI and PWI (also termed PWI/DWI- mismatch) gives an approximate measure of hypoperfused (but not yet infarcted) and potentially salvageable tissue (i.e., the penumbra). A PWI/DWI-mismatch represents an indication for thrombolysis based on potential reversibility of DWI lesions, especially if a vessel occlusion is demonstrated on MR angiography.[11] For example, if the perfusion mismatch is greater than 20% and the onset of symptoms is within a certain time window (e.g., within 6 hours for anterior circulation and within 9 hours for posterior circulation), a specific treatment decision for intervention could be made. Perfusion studies are also becoming an important diagnostic tool in a variety of other conditions, such as arteriovenous malformations, central nervous system neoplasms, epilepsy, and other developmental and degenerative central nervous system disorders.[12]

1-12 HIGH-RESOLUTION THREE-DIMENSIONAL RAPID IMAGING

Recent developments in MR hardware and pulse sequences have allowed higher-resolution imaging of labyrinthine structures, cranial nerves (Figure 1-77), perineural spread of tumors, cavernous sinus invasion, and vascular abnormalities. These sequences go by names such as CISS (constructive interference in steady-state) and FIESTA (fast imaging employing steady-state acquisition) depending on the scanner manufacturer. These newer sequences have built-in flow compensation that greatly reduces the artifact caused by CSF pulsations.[13] This sequence uses three-dimensional acquisition. The detailed anatomic information provides particular value in planning surgical interventions for both intra- and extra-axial lesions. The advantage of such sequences includes the combination of high signal levels, high contrast with the CSF, and extremely high spatial resolution. Especially for the ophthalmologist, they can be very helpful in evaluating cranial nerve pathology (e.g., oculomotor nerve schwannoma).

1-13 PARAMAGNETIC CONTRAST AGENTS

The use of contrast material for MRI improves detection of underlying pathology by demonstrating areas of blood–brain barrier breakdown. Unlike the iodinated contrast material used for CT, the contrast material for MR is a paramagnetic material called gadolinium.[14] The gadolinium paramagnetic metal ion enhances the local

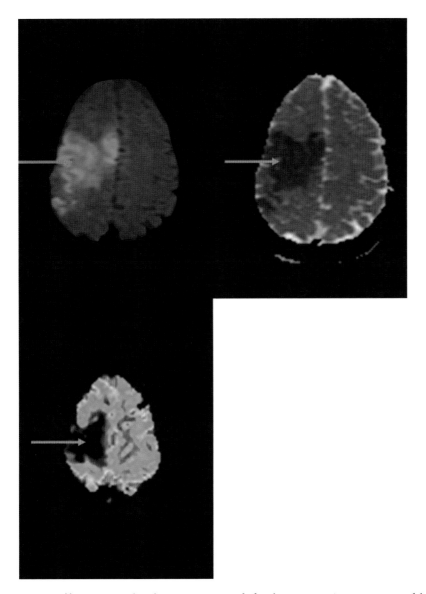

Figure 1-76. Diffusion-weighted imaging (*top left*) demonstrating an area of bright signal, which is dark on the corresponding apparent diffusion coefficient map (*top right; arrows*), consistent with an acute cerebral infarct of the right temporoparietal lobe. Perfusion-weighted imaging (*bottom*) demonstrates an area of decreased perfusion (*arrow*) with the cerebral blood volume map.

magnetic field and increases signal intensity. Gadolinium contrast agents are chelated to form a larger, more stable complex around the more toxic, free gadolinium. The stable and safe complex is excreted via the kidneys. Fortunately, unlike iodinated contrast material in CT and catheter angiography, serious side effects from gadolinium are uncommon. The most common allergic reactions are typically mild (e.g., skin rash, sweating, itching, hives, and facial swelling), but there are reports of rare

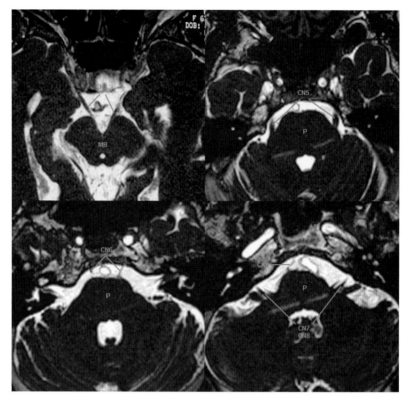

Figure 1-77. Constructive interference in steady-state MRI sequences demonstrating normal cranial nerve anatomy. CN3, third cranial nerve; CN5, fifth cranial nerve; CN6, sixth cranial nerve; CN7, seventh cranial nerve; CN8, eighth cranial nerve; MB, midbrain; P, pons.

reactions that can be severe or even fatal. Up until very recently, MRI with gadolinium was considered the "procedure of choice" in patients with renal insufficiency who required a contrast study.[14] Unfortunately, a relatively new disorder related to gadolinium contrast has emerged called nephrogenic systemic fibrosis (NSF). NSF is a fibrosing disorder seen weeks to months following gadolinium contrast administration in patients with kidney failure. NSF is characterized clinically by thickening and hardening of the skin, typically over the extremities and trunk. Although most reports relate to a specific gadolinium agent (i.e., Omniscan), the U.S. Food and Drug Administration (FDA) has issued a "black box" warning about NSF and gadolinium agents approved in the United States (e.g., Magnevist, MultiHance, ProHance, Omniscan, and OptiMark). Transmetallation (i.e., breaking the bond between the toxic metal gadolinium and the chelate [designed to block the toxic, free gadolinium ion]) might be the mechanism for NSF. The American College of Radiology (ACR) recommends against using Omniscan for patients with any stage of renal disease and caution is advised for all other gadolinium agents in patients with "moderate to severe" renal disease. Recommendations for specific glomerular filtration rate (GFR) screening are in development. Unfortunately, there is no proved therapy for NSF.[15] The main point for ophthalmologists is that, when ordering MRI with gadolinium, it is no longer an essentially "no-risk" procedure, especially in patients with renal disease. Despite these new concerns, gadolinium should probably be ordered in virtually all MR scans that are performed for a neuro-ophthalmic indication, unless there is a clear contraindication to the administration of contrast material. Patients with renal disease, diabetes, hypertension, or hepatic disease and those older than 60 years should undergo renal screening before the administration of gadolinium contrast. Gadolinium is very safe in patients without renal failure and does not produce a cross-reaction in patients with allergies to iodinated contrast or fluorescein dye.

1-14 SURFACE-COIL TECHNIQUES

In neuroimaging, surface coils may be used to evaluate superficial structures, such as the spinal cord, inner ear, and orbit. These coils are applied directly to the region of interest. The whole-body cylindrical coil within the scanner provides the excitation stimulus, and the surface coil is used only for detection. Using the surface coil to receive the RF signal is common for orbital coils, but in some magnets the head coil may be both sender and receiver of the RF signal. Because the coil covers only a small region, it allows high resolution due to an improved S/N ratio. Within the orbit, surface coils allow excellent resolution back to the apex. However, if a lesion is thought to extend through the optic foramen or the superior orbital fissure, surface coils may not be useful. In addition, surface coils are more sensitive to movement than are stationary coils and may increase movement artifact on T2WI. While excellent anatomic and pathophysiologic data concerning orbital structures have been obtained with surface coils, there are a few clinical problems for which surface coils are the only relevant solution.

1-15 MAGNETIC STRENGTH

Unlike CT, which is based on standard x-ray technology, MRI is based on detecting the signal from resonance within a large magnetic field. The static magnetic field created by the MRI scanner is expressed in Tesla (T) units. The magnetic fields of most scanners used for clinical MRI are typically 1.5 to 3.0 T (up to 9.0 T on research systems). Older MR machines, or open MR scanners, have weaker magnets (e.g., 0.3 to 1.0 T). By comparison, the earth's magnetic field is approximately 0.00005 T.[16] The MR signal is generated from the interaction of hydrogen protons (mostly in water, the H in H_2O) within the powerful magnetic field. Unlike CT, there is no radiation exposure with MRI. The number of 3.0-T scanners is increasing worldwide due to the potential technical benefits when moving from 1.5 T to 3.0 T. Weaker magnets often produce suboptimal imaging compared with larger field magnets. The benefits of larger field strength MRI include an increased S/N ratio, increased chemical shift resolution, increased sensitivity to various contrast agents, and improved vessels-versus-tissue contrast. This may translate clinically into either higher patient throughput or improved diagnostic accuracy in many neuro-ophthalmologic applications, but this is still debated.[17]

1-16 CONTRAINDICATIONS

Absolute contraindications to MRI are limited but include iron-containing intra-ocular foreign bodies, cochlear implants, and intracranial ferromagnetic vascular clips. If an intraorbital foreign body is suspected, screening anteroposterior and lateral skull films or even a limited CT scan of the orbits may be performed to look for a metallic foreign body. Cardiac pacemakers may malfunction due to repro-gramming of the unit in MR. Ventriculoperitoneal shunt–related magnetically controlled programmable valves may need to be reset after an MR study. Some patients may not be able to withstand the claustrophobic conditions under which MRI is conducted, even with sedation, but this is a relative contraindication only. The table weight capacity of newer MR scanners continues to increase (e.g., up to 550 pounds), but some older units may have lower weight limits (e.g., 350 pounds). The risks of gadolinium were previously discussed in Section 1-13.

2

Computed Tomography

The technique for computed tomography (CT) scanning was originated by Sir Godfrey N. Hounsfield at EMI (Electrical and Musical Industries) in England. As a result of his work, Sir Hounsfield was awarded the Nobel Prize in Physiology or Medicine in 1979. To understand this modality, it is necessary to begin with a brief review of x-ray and tomographic techniques.

2-1 PHYSICAL PRINCIPLES

When an x-ray is transmitted through a substance, the beam is attenuated as a function of both the atomic number of the element (or the effective atomic number of a complex structure) and the concentration of the substances forming the structure. In reality, it is the effective electron density that causes the attenuation. Increasing the energy of the x-ray leads to a decrease in attenuation. Conventional x-ray films are taken with the film alongside the patient and perpendicular to the beam. Most of the rays pass perpendicular to the film; some are scattered in other directions. Because of the thickness of the structures being filmed and the superimposition of these same structures, unwanted shadows are seen in addition to the desired image.

Tomography was invented to eliminate these undesired shadows and to concentrate on the object of interest. In this technique, the x-ray source and the film move relative to the patient during exposure. The point at which this x-ray source–film plane is pivoted is the object of interest. The desired structure remains motionless, and there is no relative movement between the film and the x-ray source.

2-2 CLINICAL IMAGING DEVICES

Hounsfield's innovation was to use a computer to improve on the technique of tomography. Initially, only axial sections were obtainable—thus, the previous term *computerized axial tomography (CAT) scanning.* An assembly was created with the x-ray detector on one side of the object to be scanned that was rigidly connected to a collimated source of x-rays on the other side. This device, the gantry, allowed the x-ray tube and the detector to rotate around the patient as a single unit and permitted the angle of incoming x-rays to be altered, creating 180 images that were 1° apart. The computer could then reconstruct the image from the data points resulting from the attenuation of the x-ray beams. These data points were represented as pixels of a numeric value, based on the attenuation noted. This attenuation seen on the two-dimensional (2D) pixel is based on the three-dimensional (3D) voxel. The original EMI matrix was an acquisition pixel grid of 80 × 80, allowing for a voxel of 3 × 3 × 13 mm. Current scanners use a grid of 512 × 512 or 1024 × 1024 pixels.

2-3 WINDOWS

The attenuation coefficient was given an arbitrary value by Hounsfield: water was set at 0 and air was set at –500. On the original scale, dense bone had a typical value of +500. Subsequently, these values were doubled, creating Hounsfield units, abbreviated HU, ranging from air at –1000 to bone at +1000. The importance of these numbers is in providing a numeric matrix from which the computer is able to yield a picture used for diagnostic purposes. The relationship of the attenuation coefficient to the entire gray scale can be displayed on a cathode-ray tube. The extremes of the scale can be modified so that differences of 1 unit or 100 units can be distinguished. This modification provides the window width, a function not possible on the conventional x-ray film. This sets the scale between black and white. The window level is the central point of the window. This can be changed to emphasize different aspects of the scanned tissue. In orbital scanning, both soft tissue and bone windows are required to assess the extent of a lesion. A central soft tissue window level is usually near 0 to 40 H, with a width of 200 to 400 H. This allows for adequate contrast between fat and air. Bone windows may have a central level between 40 and 300 H, with a width of 2400 to 3200 H. This wide window width is necessary because of the varying density of bone.

2-4 AXIAL PLANE IMAGING

The axial plane of sectioning is usually related to either the orbitomeatal line (OML) or Reid's anatomic baseline (RBL) (Figure 2-1). OML is a straight line from the lateral canthus to the center of the external auditory meatus. RBL is a line between the inferior orbital rim and the upper margin of the external auditory meatus. This so-called anthropologic baseline is 10° negative (–10°) to OML. An important angle

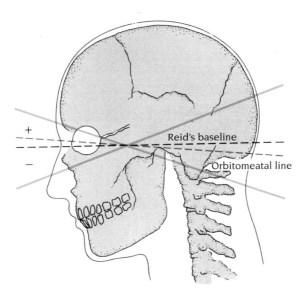

Figure 2-1. Direction of the x-ray beam in the axial plane. The orbitomeatal line extends from the lateral canthus to the center of the external auditory meatus and is the reference plane for positive (+) and negative (−) angulation. Reid's anatomic baseline extends from the inferior orbital rim to the upper margin of the external auditory meatus. Axial head scans are performed with positive angulation and may include the medulla oblongata and the base of the frontal lobe on the lowest slice; the orbit will be missed. Axial orbit scans are performed with negative angulation. Separate orbit and head sequences are usually required.

is the plane of the optic canal, which is −10° to RBL and −20° to OML. Orbits are usually scanned parallel to RBL or −10° to OML to achieve an axial-plane angle parallel to the orbital floor. For intracranial structures, angulation between 0° and +25° to OML is useful, with less positively angulated images preferred for the sellar region, the middle range preferred for the cerebral hemispheres, and the most positively angulated images preferred for the posterior fossa.

2-5 MULTIPLANAR RECONSTRUCTION

The newer multislice scanners have the ability to obtain isotropic images, so multiplanar reconstructions with good quality can be obtained. This feature eliminates the need for direct coronal images and decreases the total radiation dose for the patient.

2-6 COMPUTER ANALYSIS

CT scans can be oriented to slice or volume. Slice-oriented scanning uses single sections for diagnostic value (Figures 2-2 to Figure 2-34). Thin sections and proper alignment of the plane of scanning are crucial to achieving maximal resolution.

(*text continued on page* 79)

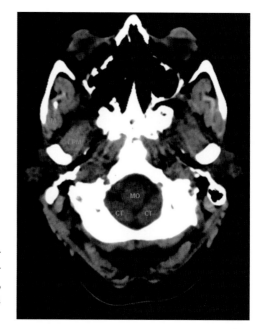

Figure 2-2. Axial CT scan near the cervicomedullary junction demonstrating normal anatomy. CT, cerebellar tonsil; LPM, lateral pterygoid muscle; MO, medulla oblongata; TM, temporalis muscle.

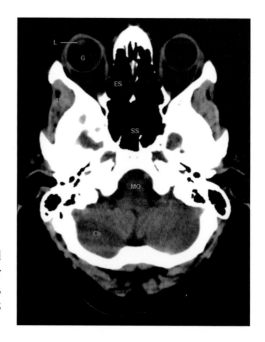

Figure 2-3. Axial CT scan of the normal medulla oblongata (MO) and cerebellar hemispheres (Cb). ES, ethmoid sinus; G, globe; L, lens; TM, temporalis muscle; SS, sphenoid sinus.

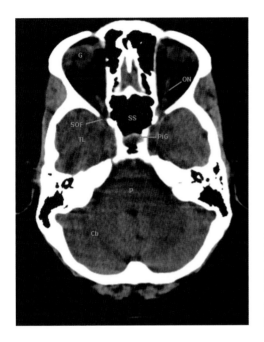

Figure 2-4. Axial CT scan demonstrating normal anatomy at the level of the pituitary gland (PiG). Cb, cerebellum; G, globe; ON, optic nerve; P, pons; SOF, superior orbital fissure; SS, sphenoid sinus; TL, temporal lobe.

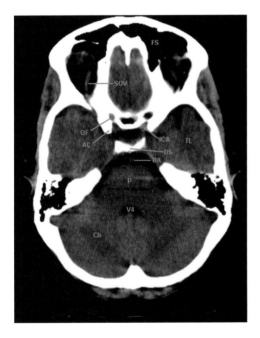

Figure 2-5. Axial CT scan demonstrating normal anatomy in the region of the sella turcica. AC, anterior clinoid process; BA, basilar artery; Cb, cerebellum; DS, dorsum sella; FS, frontal sinus; ICA, internal carotid artery; OF, optic foramen; P, pons; SOV, superior ophthalmic vein; TL, temporal lobe; V4, fourth ventricle.

65

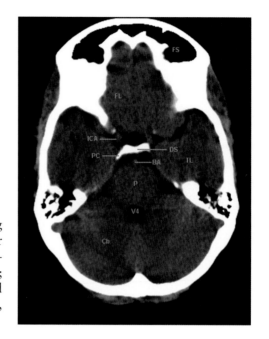

Figure 2-6. Axial CT scan demonstrating normal anatomy at the level of the upper pons (P). BA, basilar artery; Cb, cerebellum; DS, dorsum sella; FL, frontal lobe; FS, frontal sinus; ICA, internal carotid artery; PC, posterior clinoid process; TL, temporal lobe; V4, fourth ventricle.

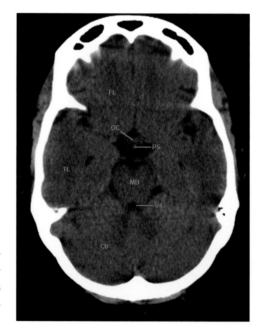

Figure 2-7. Axial CT scan demonstrating normal suprasellar anatomy. Cb, cerebellum; FL, frontal lobe; MB, midbrain; OC, optic chiasm; PS, pituitary stalk; TL, temporal lobe; V4, fourth ventricle.

66

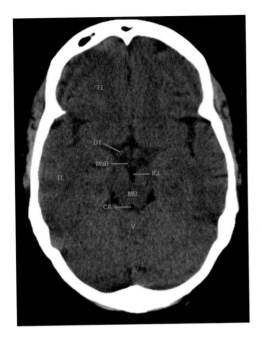

Figure 2-8. Axial CT scan at the level of the midbrain (MB) demonstrating normal anatomy. CA, cerebral aqueduct; FL, frontal lobe; ICi, interpeduncular cistern; MaB, mamillary body; OT, optic tract; TL, temporal lobe; V, vermis of cerebellum.

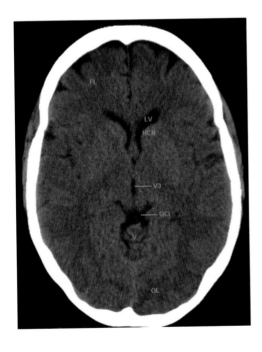

Figure 2-9. Axial CT scan at the level of the third ventricle (V3) demonstrating normal anatomy. FL, frontal lobe; HCN, head of caudate nucleus; LV, lateral ventricle; OL, occipital lobe; QCi, quadrigeminal cistern; V, vermis of cerebellum.

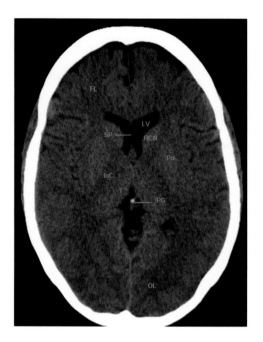

Figure 2-10. Axial CT scan demonstrating normal anatomy at the level of the internal capsule (InC). FL, frontal lobe; HCN, head of caudate nucleus; LV, lateral ventricle; OL, occipital lobe; PG, pineal gland; Pu, putamen; SP, septum pellucidum; T, thalamus.

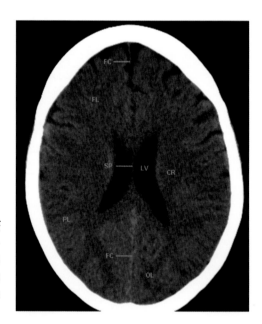

Figure 2-11. Axial CT scan at the level of the body of the lateral ventricle (LV) demonstrating normal anatomy. CR, corona radiata; FC, falx cerebri; FL, frontal lobe; OL, occipital lobe; PL, parietal lobe; SP, septum pellucidum.

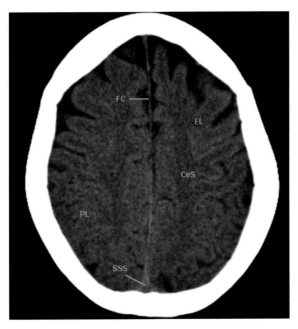

Figure 2-12. Axial CT scan demonstrating normal anatomy of the centrum semiovale (CeS). FC, falx cerebri; FL, frontal lobe; PL, parietal lobe; SSS, superior sagittal sinus.

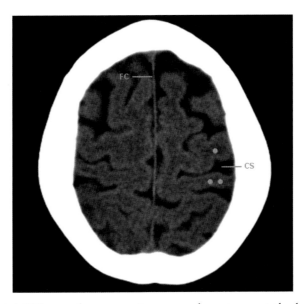

Figure 2-13. Axial CT scan demonstrating normal anatomy at the level of the upper calvarium. The central sulcus (CS) separates the precentral motor cortex (*single dot*) from the postcentral sensory cortex (*double dots*). FC, falx cerebri.

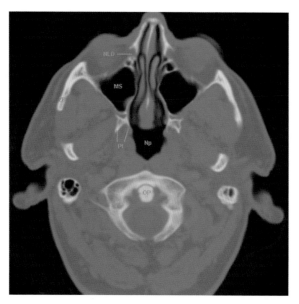

Figure 2-14. Axial bone window CT scan demonstrating normal anatomy at the level of the C1 vertebrae. MS, maxillary sinus; NLD, nasolacrimal duct; Np, nasopharynx; OP, odontoid process; Pt, pterygoid plates of sphenoid bone; ZB, zygomatic bone.

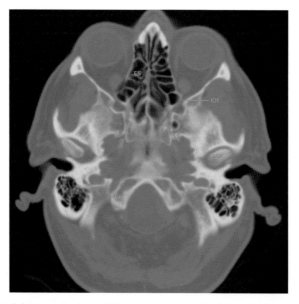

Figure 2-15. Axial bone window CT scan of the skull base demonstrating normal anatomy. ES, ethmoid sinus; IOF, inferior orbital fissure; MaC, mandibular condyle; OcC, occipital condyle.

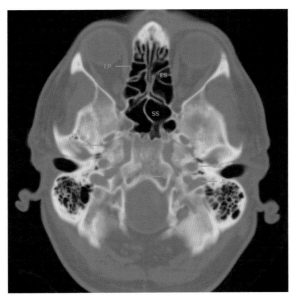

Figure 2-16. Axial bone window CT scan of the skull base demonstrating normal anatomy. C, clivus; CaC, carotid canal; ES, ethmoid sinus; FO, foramen ovale; FSp, foramen spinosum; JF, jugular foramen; LP, lamina papyracea; SS, sphenoid sinus.

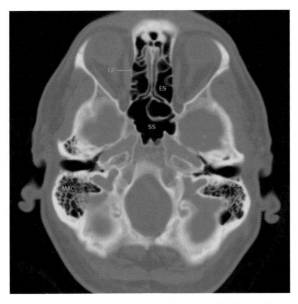

Figure 2-17. Axial bone window CT scan of the skull base demonstrating normal anatomy. C, clivus; ES, ethmoid sinus; GWS, greater wing of sphenoid bone; LP, lamina papyracea; MAC, mastoid air cells; SS, sphenoid sinus.

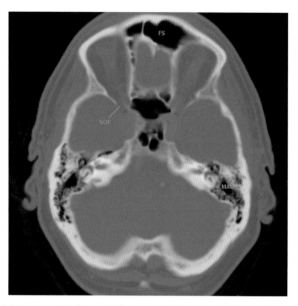

Figure 2-18. Axial bone window CT scan of the skull base demonstrating normal anatomy. FS, frontal sinus; MAC, mastoid air cells; SOF, superior orbital fissure.

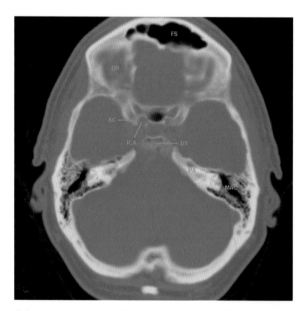

Figure 2-19. Axial bone window CT scan of the skull base demonstrating normal anatomy. AC, anterior clinoid process; DS, dorsum sella; FS, frontal sinus; ICA, internal carotid artery; MAC, mastoid air cells; OR, orbital roof; PA, petrous apex of temporal bone.

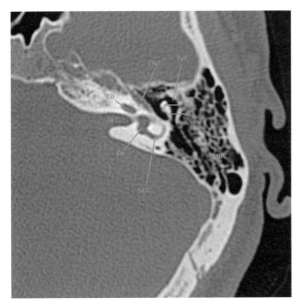

Figure 2-20. Axial bone window CT scan of the skull base at the level internal auditory canal (IAC) demonstrating normal anatomy. CN7, seventh cranial nerve; Co, cochlea; I, incus; M, malleus; MAC, mastoid air cells; ScC, semicircular canal; TyC, tympanic cavity; Ve, vestibule.

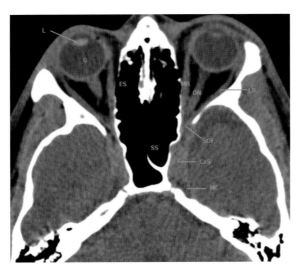

Figure 2-21. Axial CT scan of the mid-orbit demonstrating normal anatomy. CaS, cavernous sinus; ES, ethmoid sinus; G, globe; L, lens; LR, lateral rectus muscle; MC, Meckel cave; MR, medial rectus muscle; ON, optic nerve; SOF, superior orbital fissure; SS, sphenoid sinus.

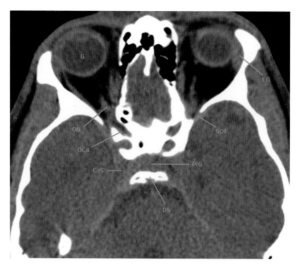

Figure 2-22. Axial CT scan of the mid-orbit demonstrating normal anatomy. CaS, cavernous sinus; DS, dorsum sella; G, globe; LG, lacrimal gland; OCa, optic canal; ON, optic nerve; PiG, pituitary gland; SOF, superior orbital fissure.

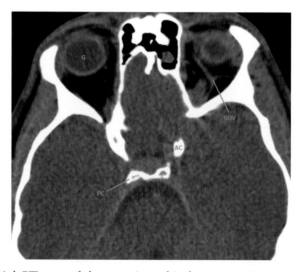

Figure 2-23. Axial CT scan of the superior orbit demonstrating normal anatomy. AC, anterior clinoid process; G, globe; PC, posterior clinoid process; SOV, superior ophthalmic vein.

74

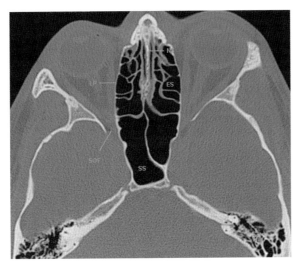

Figure 2-24. Axial bone window CT scan of the mid-orbit demonstrating normal anatomy. ES, ethmoid sinus; GWS, greater wing of sphenoid bone; LP, lamina papyracea; MAC, mastoid air cells; NS, nasal septum; PA, petrous apex of temporal bone; SOF, superior orbital fissure; SS, sphenoid sinus.

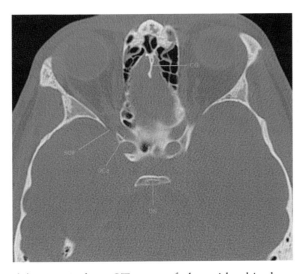

Figure 2-25. Axial bone window CT scan of the mid-orbit demonstrating normal anatomy. CG, crista galli; DS, dorsum sella; GWS, greater wing of sphenoid bone; OCa, optic canal; SOF, superior orbital fissure.

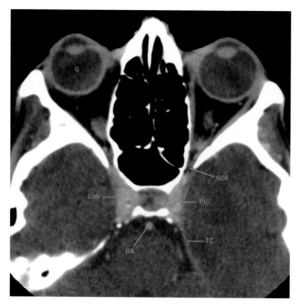

Figure 2-26. Axial postcontrast CT scan demonstrating normal cavernous sinus (CaS) anatomy. BA, basilar artery; G, globe; PiG, pituitary gland; SOF, superior orbital fissure; TC, tentorium cerebelli.

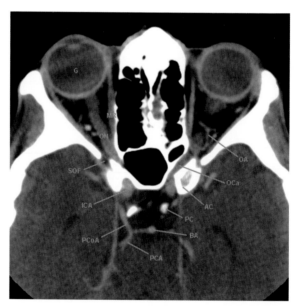

Figure 2-27. Axial postcontrast CT scan demonstrating normal anatomy of the mid-orbit. AC, anterior clinoid process; BA, basilar artery; G, globe; ICA, internal carotid artery; MR, medial rectus muscle; OA, ophthalmic artery; OCa, optic canal; ON, optic nerve; PC, posterior clinoid process; PCA, posterior cerebral artery; PCoA, posterior communicating artery; SOF, superior orbital fissure.

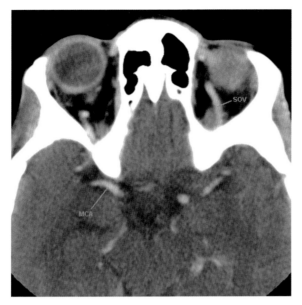

Figure 2-28. Axial postcontrast CT scan demonstrating normal anatomy of the superior orbit. MCA, middle cerebral artery; SOV, superior ophthalmic vein.

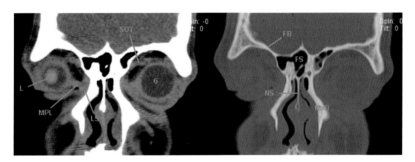

Figure 2-29. Coronal soft tissue window (*left*) and bone window (*right*) CT scans demonstrating normal anatomy at the anterior globe (G). FB, frontal bone; FS, frontal sinus; L, lens; LS, lacrimal sac; MPL, medial palpebral ligament; MxB, maxillary bone; NS, nasal septum; SOT, superior oblique muscle tendon.

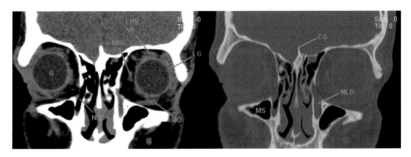

Figure 2-30. Coronal soft tissue window (*left*) and bone window (*right*) CT scans demonstrating normal anatomy at the mid-globe (G). CG, crista galli; IO, inferior oblique muscle; LG, lacrimal gland; LPS, levator palpebrae superioris muscle; MR, medial rectus muscle; MS, maxillary sinus; NLD, nasolacrimal duct; SR, superior rectus muscle.

77

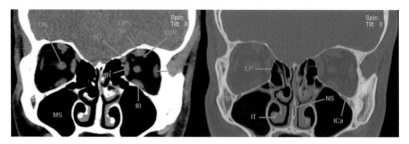

Figure 2-31. Coronal soft tissue window (*left*) and bone window (*right*) CT scans demonstrating normal orbital anatomy. FB, frontal bone; ICa, infraorbital canal; IR, inferior rectus muscle; IT, inferior turbinate; LP, lamina papyracea; LPS, levator palpebrae superioris muscle; LR, lateral rectus muscle; MR, medial rectus muscle; MS, maxillary sinus; NS, nasal septum; ON, optic nerve; SO, superior oblique muscle; SOV, superior ophthalmic vein; SR, superior rectus muscle; ZB, zygomatic bone.

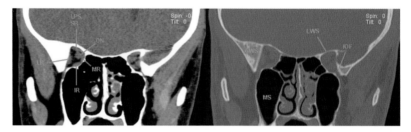

Figure 2-32. Coronal soft tissue window (*left*) and bone window (*right*) CT scans demonstrating normal orbital apex anatomy. GWS, greater wing of sphenoid bone; IR, inferior rectus muscle; IOF, interior orbital fissure; LPS, levator palpebrae superioris muscle; LR, lateral rectus muscle; LWS, lesser wing of sphenoid bone; MR, medial rectus muscle; MS, maxillary sinus; ON, optic nerve; SR, superior rectus muscle.

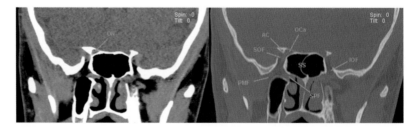

Figure 2-33. Coronal soft tissue window (*left*) and bone window (*right*) CT scans of the optic nerve (ON) within the optic canal (OCa) demonstrating normal anatomy. AC, anterior clinoid process; IOF, inferior orbital fissure; PMF, pterygomaxillary fissure; SOF, superior orbital fissure; SPF, sphenopalatine foramen; SS, sphenoid sinus.

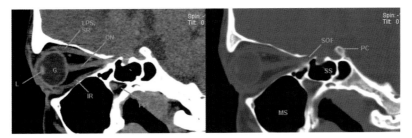

Figure 2-34. Parasagittal soft tissue window (*left*) and bone window (*right*) CT scans demonstrating normal orbital anatomy. G, globe; IR, inferior rectus muscle; L, lens; LPS, levator palpebrae superioris muscle; MS, maxillary sinus; ON, optic nerve; PC, posterior clinoid process; PPF, pterygopalatine fossa; SOF, superior orbital fissure; SR, superior rectus muscle; SS, sphenoid sinus.

Volume-oriented scanning includes overlapping adjacent thicker sections, which allows for calculations of the volume of the orbit, globe, or rectus muscles. In addition, this technique is used in plastic and reconstructive surgery to create 3D surface renderings of the bony orbit. Use of overlapping sections exposes the patient to increased radiation and causes more motion artifact.

Modern CT 3D reconstructions created with an independent workstation can produce dramatic images that demonstrate the anatomic relationships between osseous defects and sinus, orbital, or intracranial disease. In the past, clinicians would have to mentally reassemble a 3D image based on the available 2D images (e.g., axial and coronal CT images). Although modern 3D reconstruction imaging techniques can provide both aesthetically pleasing and clinically important images for surgical planning or detailed anatomic analysis, in most cases 2D imaging is sufficient.[18–20] In addition to the potential increased cost and time involved, 3D reconstruction software may smooth over pathology and may even hide subtle pathology (e.g., a minimally displaced fracture). In this setting, the 2D source images should be examined in conjunction with the 3D CT reconstructions.

2-7 CONTRAST ENHANCEMENT IN COMPUTED TOMOGRAPHY

The administration of intravenous contrast media is an important adjunct to CT scanning. Some clinical scenarios, however, do not require contrast (see later) and other clinical presentations require a noncontrast CT scan (e.g., looking for subarachnoid hemorrhage in a patient with the "worst headache of their life") (see Figure 1-72). The iodinated CT contrast material does not cross an intact blood–brain barrier and therefore there will be contrast material within the blood vessels, and if the blood–brain barrier is disrupted or absent, there will be visible contrast enhancement in the area of interest on CT.

In some cases, the contrast is unnecessary or the risk outweighs the benefit for the administration of iodinated contrast material. For example, in the diagnosis of many orbital disorders (e.g., thyroid orbitopathy or orbital fracture), there is little additional clinical need for contrast because the clinical question (e.g., "Are the extraocular muscles enlarged?" or "Is there a blowout fracture?") can be answered with a noncontrast study.

However, if intracranial extension of an orbital lesion or an inflammatory, infiltrative, or neoplastic orbital process is suspected, then administration of contrast medium may best demonstrate the lesion. The major complications following the use of iodinated contrast media are renal toxicity and allergic reactions, both of which can be life-threatening. The physician should be familiar with these problems and determine whether the patient has experienced any adverse reactions to seafood or iodine-containing contrast agents in the past.

2-8 PERFUSION COMPUTED TOMOGRAPHY

Dynamic perfusion CT (PCT) imaging is also showing progress in providing valuable information in acute stroke and tumor differentiation. Sequential images after intravenous injection of iodinated contrast are acquired using a CT scanner capable of operating in the necessary cine mode.[21] Good correlation between PCT and magnetic resonance diffusion and perfusion imaging abnormalities in acute stroke has been demonstrated.[22] Nevertheless, diffusion weighted imaging remains the sole imaging technique with the ability to assess a stroke within minutes of onset and is unlikely to be replaced by CT in the near future.[23] PCT also shows promise in distinguishing benign from malignant lesions by determining tissue perfusion characteristics.[24]

2-9 X-RAY DOSAGE

Damage to the lens may occur in the infant at doses above 750 centigray (cGy) and in the adult at doses above 2000 cGy. Standard scanning techniques result in doses of about 3 to 5 cGy in the scanned tissue, and high-resolution scanners may elevate the dosage to 10 cGy. One major concern with CT scanning is future cancer risk from the associated low-dose radiation exposure, particularly in children who require sequential or multiple imaging studies. Due to the widespread use of CT, this issue has become a public health concern.[25] Further work is needed in this area, but a proposed action plan to address radiation exposure risk was published by the American College of Radiology.[26,27]

3

Angiography and Other Specialized Imaging

Ophthalmologists should be aware of other special imaging techniques for assessing vascular lesions. The current widespread use of magnetic resonance (MR) angiography (MRA) and computed tomography (CT) angiography (CTA) has significantly reduced the use of invasive catheter angiography in the initial evaluation of vascular disease (Figures 3-1 to 3-5). Catheter angiography shows iodinated contrast-filled vessels without interference from the background (digital subtraction angiography). The background images of the normal brain are taken as "mask images" and then "subtracted" from the images after injection of contrast material. Postprocessing, such as windowing and filtering, can improve the final images. Technical advances have allowed three-dimensional rotational angiography reconstructions, which eliminate the need for multiple oblique views and thereby decrease the amount of contrast needed and the duration of radiation exposure. These three-dimensional reconstructions also have the advantage of being better able to delineate the neck of an aneurysm and can provide a more accurate measure of the coil size needed for embolization.[15] The morbidity and mortality of modern catheter angiography have been declining with better techniques, but there remains a significant, albeit small (≈1%), risk of severe complication (e.g., ischemic stroke).[28,29]

3-1 MAGNETIC RESONANCE AND COMPUTED TOMOGRAPHY ANGIOGRAPHY AND VENOGRAPHY

The technique of MRA relies on the flow-sensitive nature of the MR signal. In conventional MR imaging (MRI), the fast-moving blood appears dark on all sequences as a "flow void." There are two basic types of MRA: (1) time-of-flight (TOF) MRA

(*text continued on page 84*)

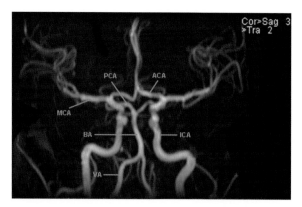

Figure 3-1. MR angiography (MRA) demonstrating a normal anterior view of the circle of Willis. ACA, anterior cerebral artery; BA, basilar artery; ICA, internal carotid artery; MCA, middle cerebral artery; PCA, posterior cerebral artery; VA, vertebral artery.

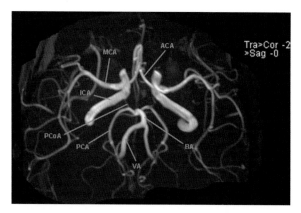

Figure 3-2. MR angiography (MRA) demonstrating a normal superior view of the circle of Willis. ACA, anterior cerebral artery; BA, basilar artery; ICA, internal carotid artery; MCA, middle cerebral artery; PCA, posterior cerebral artery; PCoA, posterior communicating artery; VA, vertebral artery.

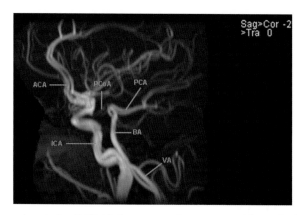

Figure 3-3. MR angiography (MRA) demonstrating a normal lateral view of the circle of Willis. ACA, anterior cerebral artery; BA, basilar artery; ICA, internal carotid artery; PCA, posterior cerebral artery; PCoA, posterior communicating artery; VA, vertebral artery.

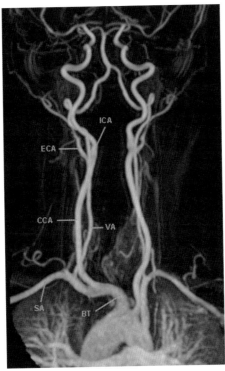

Figure 3-4. MR angiography (MRA) of the neck (anterior view) demonstrating normal anatomy. AA, aortic arch; BT, brachiocephalic trunk; CCA, common carotid artery; ECA, external carotid artery; ICA, internal carotid artery; SA, subclavian artery; VA, vertebral artery.

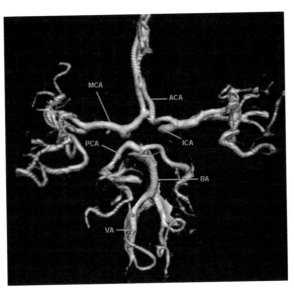

Figure 3-5. CT angiography (CTA) demonstrating normal anatomy of the circle of Willis. ACA, anterior cerebral artery; BA, basilar artery; ICA, internal carotid artery; MCA, middle cerebral artery; PCA, posterior cerebral artery; VA, vertebral artery.

and (2) phase contrast (PC) MRA. Both TOF and PC MRA can acquire data using either a two-dimensional (2D) or a three-dimensional (3D) scan. The 2D MRA acquires data slices individually and produces contiguous or overlapping data sets, while the 3D MRA technique acquires the data in a block of tissue volume. The 2D TOF MRA is more sensitive to slow flow (e.g., venous flow), but the 3D MRA technique produces thinner MRA slices and has a higher signal-to-noise ratio. The addition of contrast material enhances the 3D MRA acquisition and optimizes visualization of possible dural venous sinus disease and is also useful in evaluation of carotid stenosis. PC MRA uses gradients to induce phase shifts in flowing blood. Both PC and TOF MRA studies must undergo postprocessing to produce an MRA image that resembles a conventional catheter angiogram. We believe that TOF MRA is a more robust technique than PC MRA for evaluating vascular abnormalities of interest to ophthalmologists (e.g., aneurysms, arteriovenous malformations [AVMs]). Regardless of which technique is used, the neuroradiologist should examine the actual source images.

MRA has some advantages over CTA; these include the lack of ionizing radiation exposure, a less nephrotoxic contrast material (i.e., gadolinium versus iodinated contrast), increased signal-to-noise ratio, and easier postprocessing techniques. The advantages of CTA over MRA are increased spatial resolution, a technically easier and faster study to acquire, and less motion artifact. The critical advantage of MRA in the evaluation of a third nerve palsy is that a single MRI/MRA combination study is likely easier to obtain than two separate imaging studies (i.e., MRI and a CTA). Because the conventional MR scan is a superior study to a CT scan for assessing nonaneurysmal causes of third nerve palsy, the combination of MRI and MRA rather than MRI with CTA is likely to be the preferred imaging technique by an ophthalmologist for a patient with a third nerve palsy.[29] The sensitivity and specificity of both MRA and CTA for ophthalmic indications are probably equivalent. However, CTA may be superior to MRA in some instances, and at some institutions, depending on the amount of experience with this technique, a CTA might be performed first, followed by a contrast MRI if the CTA is negative.

One of the "highest stakes" situations for which the ophthalmologist might need to decide between invasive (catheter angiogram) versus noninvasive (MR or CT) angiography is in the evaluation of third cranial nerve palsy. Table 3-1 describes the use of MRA and CTA in third nerve palsy.[28,29] For patients with pupil-involving or partial third nerve palsy, MRA or CTA offers a less invasive method of evaluation than catheter angiography for detecting aneurysms (Figure 3-6). The published sensitivity of both MRA and CTA in detecting an aneurysm causing a third nerve palsy is as high as 98% but is not 100%.[28–32] Thus, catheter angiography may still be required if the pretest (i.e., MRA or CTA) likelihood for harboring an aneurysm is high and even if the posttest likelihood of aneurysm (i.e., negative MRA or CTA) is moderate to high. The size of an aneurysm needed to produce a third nerve palsy would likely be within the detection limit of most scanners used for MRA and CTA (usually ≥5 mm). Newer machines and improved techniques have increased resolution sufficiently to reliably detect aneurysms as small

Table 3-1. Recommended Neuroimaging for Acute Isolated Third Cranial Nerve Palsy Based on Degree of Internal and External Dysfunction and Risk of Aneurysm

Isolated Third Nerve Palsy	Complete External Dysfunction	Incomplete External Dysfunction	No External Dysfunction
Complete internal dysfunction	Highest risk CTA then MRI/MRA Angiography may still be needed*	Highest risk CTA then MRI/MRA Angiography may still be needed*	Minimal if any risk No imaging for aneurysm required
Incomplete internal dysfunction	Uncertain but probably low risk CTA then MRI/MRA Consider angiography*	Moderate risk CTA then MRI/MRA Consider angiography*	Minimal if any risk No imaging for aneurysm required
No internal dysfunction	Low risk Initial observation† MRI/MRA or CTA if no improvement	Uncertain risk CTA then MRI/MRA Consider angiography*	Not applicable

Modified from Lee AG, Hayman LA, Brazis PW. The evaluation of isolated third nerve palsy revisited: an update on the evolving role of magnetic resonance, computed tomography, and catheter angiography. *Surv Ophthalmol.* 2002;47:137–157.

CTA, computed tomography angiography; MRA, magnetic resonance angiography; MRI, magnetic resonance imaging.

*Catheter angiography should still be considered for patients in whom the risk of aneurysm is higher than the risk of angiography. Catheter angiography is recommended if (1) worsening of extraocular muscle or iris sphincter impairment continues beyond 14 days, (2) iris sphincter impairment progresses to anisocoria >1 mm,[33] (3) no recovery of function occurs within 12 weeks, or (4) signs of aberrant regeneration develop.[28]

†Vasculopathic patients (e.g., hypertension or diabetes) with complete external dysfunction and no internal dysfunction may be observed for improvement without neuroimaging, as it is very likely to be due to an ischemic third nerve palsy. Patients without vasculopathic risk factors or vasculopathic patients who do not improve or who progress over a few months' time should undergo a neuroimaging study (MRI with MRA or CTA).

as 2 to 3 mm.[32] However, because the "gold standard" evaluation for a cerebral aneurysm remains catheter angiography, we recommend catheter angiography be considered for high suspicion cases even with a negative MRA or CTA (e.g., poor MRA or CTA visualization of the posterior communicating artery, incomplete or poor quality study, painful pupil-involving third nerve palsy, other risk factors for aneurysm, subarachnoid hemorrhage).

For the ophthalmologist, other indications for ordering CTA or MRA include evaluation of an AVM, a dural or carotid cavernous fistula, and suspected carotid artery disease (e.g., carotid dissection, stenosis, or occlusion). When comparing contrast enhanced MRA with digital subtraction angiography for evaluation of carotid stenosis, MRA had a pooled sensitivity of 95% and specificity of 90%.[34] CTA has a similar sensitivity and specificity to MRA, and both have a slightly higher sensitivity and specificity than Doppler ultrasonography.[35] Finally, the use of MRA or CTA may also be helpful in patients with hemispheric transient ischemic attacks, homonymous hemianopsias, transient monocular visual loss (i.e., amaurosis fugax), or completed cortical strokes.

The major ophthalmic indication for performing a venogram is to exclude dural venous sinus thrombosis in patients presenting with papilledema from increased

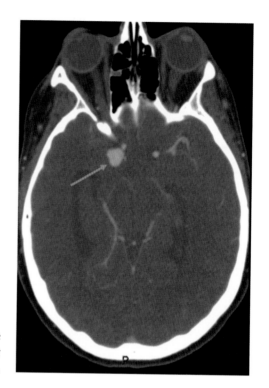

Figure 3-6. CT angiogram (CTA) source image demonstrating a right posterior communicating artery aneurysm (arrow).

intracranial pressure. Symptoms of cerebral venous sinus thrombosis may mimic those of idiopathic intracranial hypertension. A standard head CT can often show direct and indirect signs of venous thrombosis, but in about one third of cases it is normal.[36] Nonenhanced MRI of the brain is more sensitive than noncontrast CT for showing parenchymal abnormalities and the presence of intraluminal thrombus in the sinus. Other MR findings include the absence of a flow void and the presence of altered signal intensity in the thrombosed sinus.[37] A number of venographic techniques have been developed to better define sinus anatomy. These include PC MR venography (PC MRV), unenhanced TOF MR venography (TOF MRV), contrast-enhanced MRV (Figure 3-7), and CT venography (CTV). Contrast-enhanced MRV reduces the artifact that is commonly seen with non-contrast PC MRV (e.g., distal transverse or sigmoid sinus flow reduction mimicking stenosis or occlusion).[38–40] Depiction of the dural sinuses and small-vessel visualization is also improved with contrast-enhanced MRV compared with TOF MRV.[41] CTV is another method for detecting cerebral venous thrombosis that is both rapid and widely available.[37] CTV can provide very detailed imaging of the venous system, which is superior to TOF MRV and is at least as accurate for detecting thrombosis.[42] Disadvantages to CTV include the use of iodinated contrast material, ionizing radiation exposure, and difficulty in reconstructing maximum intensity projection (MIP) images due to problems subtracting bone adjacent to the venous sinuses.[37] Our preferred technique for evaluating cerebral venous sinus thrombosis is a precontrast and postcontrast MRI with a contrast-enhanced MRV (Figure 3-8).

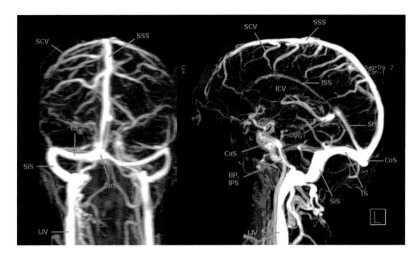

Figure 3-7. Anterior (*left*) and lateral (*right*) view of normal cerebral venous anatomy using contrast-enhanced MR venography (MRV). BP, basilar venous plexus; CaS, cavernous sinus; CoS, confluence of sinuses; ICV, internal cerebral vein; IJV, internal jugular vein; IPS, inferior petrosal sinus; ISS, inferior sagittal sinus; SCV, superficial cortical vein; SiS, sigmoid sinus; SSS, superior sagittal sinus; StS, straight sinus; TS, transverse sinus; VG, vein of Galen.

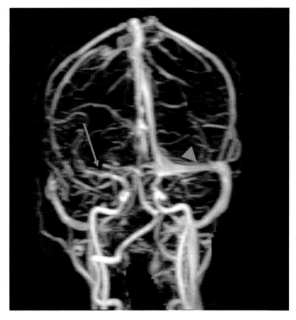

Figure 3-8. Contrast-enhanced MR venography (MRV) demonstrating poor filling of the right transverse sinus (*arrow*) compared with the normal left transverse sinus (*arrowhead*).

3-2 MAGNETIC RESONANCE SPECTROSCOPY

MR spectroscopy (MRS) is another evolving MR technique that is based on detecting various proton MR spectra.[43] The commonly measured metabolites in MRS include N-acetyl-aspartate (NAA), creatine and phosphocreatine, choline-containing phospholipids, and lactate. Other metabolites like glutamate, glutamine, gamma-aminobutyric acid, myoinositol, and fatty acids can also be assessed. Although an ophthalmologist is unlikely to be ordering MRS, a brief description of the technology might be useful. NAA is a neuronal and axonal integrity marker, and a reduction of the NAA peak on MRS is a marker for neuronal/axonal dysfunction (e.g., certain tumors have no NAA, such as meningiomas or metastases) or markedly decreased NAA (e.g., glioblastoma multiforme, metastases). Creatine may be elevated in hypometabolic states (e.g., ischemia or certain tumors like gliomatosis cerebri) and decreased in hypermetabolic states. Choline is a component of cell membranes, and increased choline might suggest increased membrane synthesis (e.g., active proliferating or a solid, hypercellular tumor). Because the creatine level often remains stable even in disease states, creatine can be used as a control for MRS with levels of other metabolites expressed as a ratio to creatine (e.g., increased choline/creatine ratio in certain brain tumors). The normal brain derives energy from aerobic metabolism of glucose and, therefore, a significant lactate peak on MRS might indicate anaerobic metabolism (e.g., metabolic disturbances, ischemia, trauma, and tumors). Lipid and myoinositol are markers of gliosis and myelin damage and might be elevated in specific disease states. The spectrum of MRS applications in neuro-ophthalmology has been expanding and includes differentiating ischemic, neoplastic, demyelinating, radiation necrosis, inflammatory, and mitochondrial disorders.

3-3 FUNCTIONAL MAGNETIC RESONANCE IMAGING

As opposed to structural imaging studies (e.g., MRI and CT), functional imaging studies show information about the physiology and metabolic function of brain. These functional studies might be particularly useful when structural imaging appears normal despite clinical findings that suggest underlying brain dysfunction. Functional MR imaging (fMRI) is based on changes in the T2 signal due to deoxyhemoglobin. The signal change of blood oxygenation level–dependent (BOLD) mechanisms can be imaged on fMRI. Localized increases in neuronal activity from task-related brain activation produce increased cerebral blood flow and decreased deoxyhemoglobin, and this can be imaged with fMRI. Presurgical mapping of brain function, including localization of visual functions, has provided new insights into brain physiology. Functional MRI has many potential advantages because it is noninvasive, does not require the injection of contrast agents, and has relatively high spatial and temporal resolution. It can be repeated many times during the course of a longitudinal study, such as in clinical drug trials.[44,45] There are few clinical indications for which the general ophthalmologist would require fMRI.

Other functional imaging studies that have increasing application in ophthalmology are positron emission tomography (PET) and single-photon emission computed tomography (SPECT). Both PET and SPECT use radiolabeled molecules to image local metabolic changes (e.g., regional blood flow and glucose metabolism). PET has superior sensitivity and tissue resolution compared with SPECT but is more expensive and less widely available. Because PET scanning can image the whole body or a single organ, it has found use in the evaluation of systemic sarcoidosis and in the search for occult neoplasms. For example, it might be useful in patients with suspected sarcoidosis in whom a suitable biopsy site is not readily apparent. Less common potential applications for PET and SPECT include the evaluation of cerebral toxicity (e.g., cyclosporine-related cerebral blindness), intracranial or systemic neoplasms (e.g., primary or metastatic disease), inflammatory disease (e.g., sarcoidosis), radiation necrosis, stroke, degenerative disorders, epilepsy, movement disorders, and migraine. Finally, another ophthalmic application for PET is in assessment of patients with organic homonymous hemianopsias or cortical blindness (e.g., carbon monoxide poisoning, visual variant Alzheimer disease). In these cases, the traditional structural imaging may show no lesion but PET might show occipital hypometabolism ("cold") or hypermetabolism ("hot").[46–49]

4

Ordering and Interpreting Images

The specific indications for obtaining imaging in particular disease entities are beyond the scope of this volume. Images should be ordered after a complete history has been taken, a thorough examination performed, and a differential diagnosis entertained. In some conditions, several clinical examinations of the patient may be more valuable than obtaining imaging studies after the first visit. The better defined the differential diagnosis, the more appropriate will be the imaging, enhancing the value of the scanning to the patient. Both magnetic resonance imaging (MRI) and computed tomography (CT) techniques should be used for any situation where they may be complementary, and they should be extended or repeated if necessary to obtain the required information.

4-1 SELECTION OF TECHNIQUE

In general, a CT scan is not as sensitive or specific as an MR image for neuro-ophthalmic indications (e.g., intracranial process) or for orbital processes with possible intracranial extension. CT scanning is probably sufficient, however, for many strictly orbital conditions (e.g., thyroid eye disease [Figure 4-1], idiopathic orbital inflammation [Figure 4-2], and orbital tumors [Figure 4-3]) and may be superior to (e.g., orbital fracture, bone disease, calcification) or complementary to (e.g., fibrous dysplasia, optic nerve sheath meningioma, concomitant sinus disease, suspected foreign body) an MR image. Typically, however, MR imaging (MRI) is the neuroimaging study of choice for almost all other neuro-ophthalmic indications unless there is a contraindication. MRI is superior to CT for soft tissue discrimination of intracranial anatomy (e.g., meninges, cavernous sinus, posterior fossa, and dural venous sinuses) and pathology.

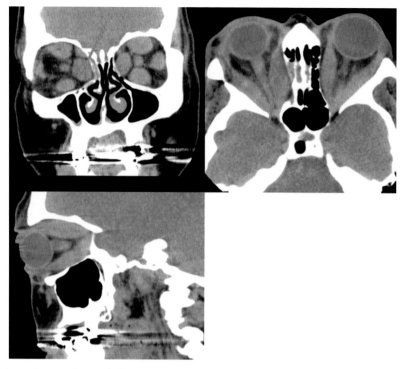

Figure 4-1. Coronal (*top left*), axial (*top right*), and sagittal (*bottom*) CT scans demonstrating enlarged extraocular muscles bilaterally, especially the medial rectus muscles (*arrows*), consistent with thyroid eye disease.

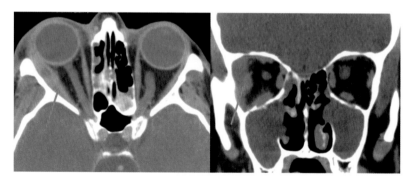

Figure 4-2. Axial (*left*) and coronal (*right*) CT scans of the orbit demonstrating irregular enlargement of the right lateral rectus muscle (*arrows*) in a patient with idiopathic orbital inflammation.

As mentioned, however, there are specific circumstances where CT may be superior or complementary to MRI. The most prominent example is that CT is better for demonstrating calcification and bone but CT (often in conjunction with MRI) is helpful in the differential diagnosis of many disorders that affect both the orbit and brain (e.g., meningioma), bone (e.g., primary bony tumors, bone erosion or destruction, or lytic lesions), or the adjacent sinuses or skull base (e.g., orbital,

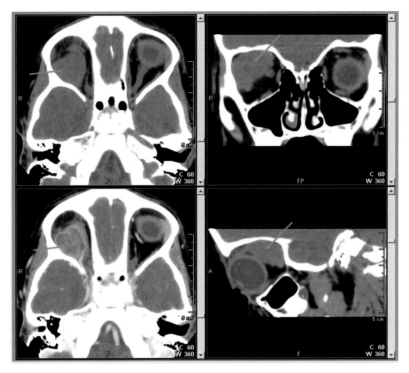

Figure 4-3. Axial precontrast (*top left*), coronal precontrast (*top right*), axial postcontrast (*bottom left*), and parasagittal precontrast (*bottom right*) CT scans demonstrating an irregular enhancing mass (*arrows*) in the superior orbit of a child consistent with rhabdomyosarcoma.

maxillofacial, calvarial or skull base fracture, hyperostosis of bone associated with meningiomas [Figure 4-4], fibrous dysplasia, sphenoid wing agenesis in neurofibromatosis-1, craniosynostosis syndromes, sinusitis or sinus tumors, clival lesions).

The presence of calcification that might be better seen on a CT scan, however, is important in the evaluation of specific ophthalmic and neuro-ophthalmic conditions (e.g., optic nerve head drusen,[50] craniopharyngioma, meningioma, retinoblastoma [Figure 4-5], dystrophic calcification, calcified intracranial tumors). A noncontrast CT scan is also the first-line neuroimaging study for hyperdensity of acute hemorrhage (e.g., orbital, subdural, subarachnoid, intraventricular, or intraparenchymal hemorrhage (e.g., associated with trauma, tumor, stroke, or ruptured aneurysm)).

In addition, CT scanning is generally easier and faster to perform for the patient than MRI and is often more widely available in the emergent and community setting. Thus, CT scanning is usually preferred in the "after hours," urgent, or emergent imaging setting (e.g., emergency department visit, acute head or orbital trauma, acute stroke, intracranial or intraorbital bleed or abscess, pituitary apoplexy, or intracranial shunt malfunction). Following the emergent CT scan, a follow-up MR study might still be necessary due to the superior soft tissue resolution of MRI.

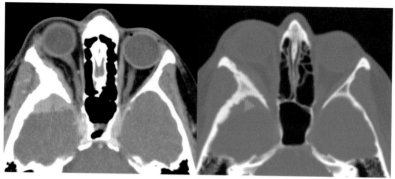

Figure 4-4. Axial soft tissue window postcontrast CT scansof the head (*left*) demonstrating an extraaxial mass involving the sphenoid bone with intraorbital extension and involvement of the lateral orbit and lateral rectus muscle consistent with a meningioma (*arrow*). The bone window CT view of the sphenoid bone (*right*) demonstrates hyperostosis of the bone (*arrowhead*), which is commonly associated with meningiomas in this location.

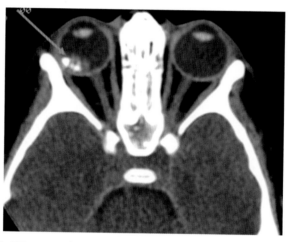

Figure 4-5. Axial CT scan of the orbit demonstrating hyperdense signal (*arrow*) in a posterior segment intraocular mass suggestive of a calcified tumor—in this case, a retinoblastoma.

The most important clinical scenarios for an ophthalmologist to consider an urgent or emergent orbital or head CT scan include the following:

1. Acute orbital trauma (e.g., suspected orbital fracture [Figure 4-6], penetrating or perforating open globe injury [Figure 4-7], orbital hematoma, metallic or wooden foreign bodies,[51,52] or traumatic optic neuropathy)
2. Acute-onset proptosis (e.g., orbital cellulitis or orbital abscess, idiopathic orbital inflammation, thyroid orbitopathy with compressive optic neuropathy or vision-threatening proptosis, postsurgical or spontaneous retrobulbar hemorrhage, rupture or bleeding from an intraorbital or carotid cavernous sinus lesion [Figure 4-8])

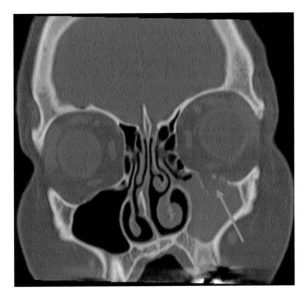

Figure 4-6. Coronal bone window CT scan demonstrating a left orbital floor fracture (*arrow*).

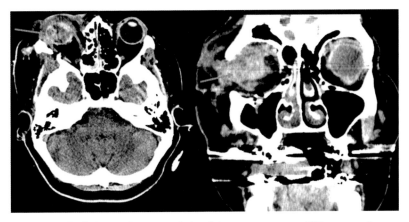

Figure 4-7. Axial (*left*) and coronal (*right*) noncontrast CT scans demonstrating disruption of the globe wall and intraocular contents (*arrows*) consistent with an open globe injury.

3. Acute bitemporal hemianopsia (e.g., pituitary apoplexy)*
4. Acute homonymous hemianopsia or cortical blindness (e.g., acute stroke, acute hemorrhage from tumor or arteriovenous lesion)*
5. Acute, severe headache (i.e., "worst headache of my life") with or without acute third nerve palsy (e.g., subarachnoid hemorrhage due to ruptured intracranial aneurysm [see Figure 1-72], pituitary apoplexy)

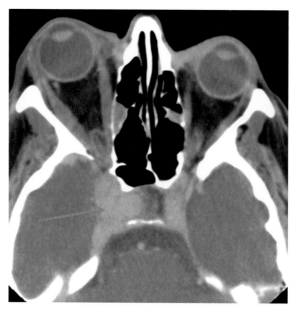

Figure 4-8. Axial postcontrast CT scan of the orbits demonstrating proptosis of the right globe. There is asymmetric fullness and enhancement in the right cavernous sinus (*arrow*) due to a carotid-cavernous fistula.

6. Acute papilledema (e.g., to rule out intracranial tumor or bleed in the emergent setting)*
7. Acute visual loss, headache, or diplopia especially in a patient unable to undergo MRI*

Although MRI is superior to CT for most ophthalmic indications, there are both relative and absolute contraindications to performing MRI for which CT might then be the alternate imaging choice (e.g., severe claustrophobia, marked obesity exceeding table weight limit, cochlear implant, ferromagnetic aneurysm clip, pacemaker, or other metallic foreign body). We emphasize that CT and MRI are complementary studies and the use of CT or MRI is not mutually exclusive. This is particularly true for lesions that have both soft tissue and osseous changes (e.g., sphenoid wing meningioma with hyperostosis or orbital dermoid cyst [Figure 4-9]).

The ophthalmologist should communicate the clinical findings, topographical localization, differential diagnosis, and urgency of the imaging request to the neuroradiologist on the requisition. Wolintz et al. described common requisition errors when ordering ophthalmologic studies.[53] These authors described the following prescriptive errors: "1) failure to apply a dedicated study, 2) inappropriate use of

---

*In most of these conditions (except perhaps orbital cellulitis or orbital trauma), follow-up MRI will still probably be necessary after emergent CT has been performed.

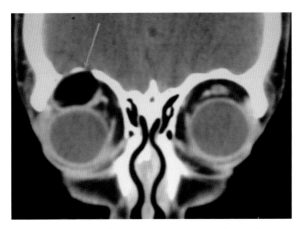

Figure 4-9. Coronal CT scan of the orbit demonstrating a hypodense mass with a hyperdense rim in the superior orbit (*arrow*) consistent with an orbital dermoid with internal fat density.

a dedicated study, 3) omission of intravenous contrast, and 4) omission of specialized sequences." The following interpretive errors were also reported: "1) failure to detect the lesion because of misleading clinical information, 2) rejection of a clinical diagnosis because an expected imaging abnormality was absent, 3) assumption that a striking imaging abnormality accounted for the clinical abnormality, and 4) failure to consider the lack of clinical specificity of imaging abnormalities."[53] Table 4-1 lists the common ophthalmic indications for ordering an imaging study, and Table 4-2 summarizes our recommendations for contacting the neuroradiologist to discuss the clinical indications, differential diagnosis, topographical localization, and urgency of the study.

4-2 INTERPRETING IMAGES

As in other disciplines, interpreting CT and MRI scans requires practice and a systematic approach. It is important to review the preliminary data provided on the scan. This includes the patient's name and age, date of scan, technique, whether contrast enhancement was used, slice thickness, and right–left orientation. On CT scans, the window width and center are provided and the order of scans is usually listed by image number. On MR images, TR, TE, and TI should be reviewed to assess the weighting of the image. In addition, the ACQ or NEX, matrix, and FOV are provided. Slice location is usually centered around a point designated as zero, with the initial scans shown as negative with regard to the zero position. Standard convention is to scan from inferior to superior in the axial plane and from anterior to posterior in the coronal plane. The sagittal-plane convention is the most variable.

Table 4-1. Neuro-ophthalmic Indications and Recommended Imaging Study

Clinical Indication	Preferred Imaging Study	Contrast Material	Comment
Optic nerve drusen	CT scan of the orbit may show calcification.	Not necessary	Orbital ultrasound is less costly and more sensitive than a CT scan for optic disc head drusen.[49]
Bilateral optic disc swelling	MRI head (with MRV) CT scan might be first-line study in emergent setting.	Yes	Consider concomitant contrast MRV to exclude venous sinus thrombosis (see Figure 3–8), especially in atypical cases of pseudotumor cerebri who are thin, male, or elderly.
Transient monocular visual loss (amaurosis fugax) due to ischemia	MRA or CTA of neck for carotid stenosis or dissection	Depends on clinical situation	Carotid Doppler study might be first line and may still require follow-up catheter angiography.
Demyelinating optic neuritis	MRI head and orbit	Yes (enhancing lesions suggest acute disease)	FLAIR to look for demyelinating white matter lesions. MRI has prognostic significance for development of multiple sclerosis.
Inflammatory, infiltrative, or compressive optic neuropathy	MRI head and orbit	Yes	Fat suppression to exclude intraorbital optic nerve enhancement (see Figure 1–69). CT is superior in traumatic optic neuropathy for canal fractures.
Junctional scotoma (i.e., optic neuropathy in one eye and superotemporal field loss in fellow eye)	MRI head (attention to sella)	Yes	Junctional lesions are typically mass lesions.
Bitemporal hemianopsia	MRI head (attention to chiasm and sella) (Figures 4-10 and 4-11)	Yes	Consider CT of sella if an emergent scan is needed (e.g., pituitary or chiasmal apoplexy) or if imaging for calcification (e.g., meningioma or craniopharyngioma or aneurysm).

Homonymous hemianopsia	MRI head	Yes	Retrochiasmal pathway DWI may be useful if acute ischemic infarct (see Figure 1–74) or PRES (see Figure 1–75). If structural imaging negative and organic loss, consider functional imaging like PET.
Cortical visual loss or visual association cortex (e.g., cerebral achromatopsia, alexia, prosopagnosia, simultagnosia, optic ataxia, Balint syndrome)	MRI head	Yes	Retrochiasmal pathway Consider DWI in ischemic infarct. If structural imaging negative and organic loss, consider functional imaging (e.g., PET, SPECT, or MRS).
Third, fourth, sixth nerve palsy or cavernous sinus syndrome	MRI head with attention to the skull base Isolated vasculopathic cranial neuropathies may not require initial imaging. See Table 3–1 for third nerve palsy evaluation with MRA or CTA.	Yes	Rim calcification in aneurysm, calcification in tumors, and hyperostosis may be better seen on CT.
Internuclear ophthalmoplegia (INO), supranuclear or nuclear gaze palsies, dorsal midbrain syndrome, skew deviation	MRI head (brainstem)	Yes	Rule out demyelinating or other brainstem lesion. Include a FLAIR sequence.
Nystagmus	MRI brainstem	Yes	Localize nystagmus.
Hemifacial spasm	MRI brainstem (with or without MRA)	Yes	Facial nerve compression at root exit zone

(continued)

Table 4-1. *Continued*

Clinical Indication	Preferred Imaging Study	Contrast Material	Comment
Horner syndrome: preganglionic	MRI head and neck to second thoracic vertebra (T2) in chest with neck MRA*	Yes	Rule out lateral medullary infarct, brachial plexus injury, apical lung neoplasm, carotid dissection, etc.
Horner syndrome: postganglionic	MRI head and neck to level of superior cervical ganglion (C4 level) with MRA neck[†]	Yes	Rule out carotid dissection. Isolated postganglionic lesions are often benign.
Thyroid eye disease	CT or MRI of orbit	Iodinated contrast may interfere with evaluation and treatment of systemic thyroid disease.	Bone anatomy is better seen on a CT scan, especially if orbital decompression is being considered (see Figure 4-1).
Orbital cellulitis and orbital disease secondary to sinus disease	CT orbit and sinuses	Depends on clinical situation	MRI and/or CT with CTA may be useful adjunct to a CT alone, especially if possible concomitant cavernous sinus thrombosis is present.
Idiopathic orbital inflammation	CT or MRI of orbit (with fat suppression)	Yes	Beware fat-suppression artifact.
Orbital tumor (e.g., proptosis or enophthalmos, gaze-evoked visual loss)	CT or MRI of orbit	Yes	Include head imaging if lesion could extend intracranially. MRI with contrast is superior at determining intracranial extent of primary optic nerve tumors (e.g., optic nerve glioma or sheath meningioma) (Figures 4-12 and 4-13). CT scan may be superior if looking for hyperostosis or calcification.

Orbital trauma (e.g., orbital fracture, subperiosteal hematoma, orbital foreign body, orbital emphysema)	CT scan of orbit with direct coronal	Not generally necessary	CT is superior to MRI for bone fractures.
Traumatic optic neuropathy	CT of optic canal (thin sections)	Not generally necessary	CT is superior for visualizing fracture or bone fragment.
Carotid-cavernous sinus or dural fistula (e.g., orbital bruit, arterialization of conjunctival and episcleral vessels, glaucoma)	CT or MRI of head and orbit (with contrast-enhanced MRA)	Yes	CT or MRI may show enlarged superior ophthalmic vein. May require catheter angiogram for final diagnosis and therapy. Color flow Doppler studies may be useful for detecting reversal of orbital venous flow.

Modified from Reference 54.

CT, computed tomography; CTA, computed tomography angiography; DWI, diffusion weighted imaging; FLAIR, fluid attenuation inversion recovery; MRA, magnetic resonance angiography; MRI, magnetic resonance imaging; MRS, magnetic resonance spectroscopy; MRV, magnetic resonance venography; PET, positron emission tomography; PRES, posterior reversible encephalopathy syndrome; SPECT, single photon emission computed tomography.

*When the presumed lesion is in the lung, mediastinum, or anterior aspect of the neck, contrast-enhanced axial CT may be sufficient for localization.[55,56]

†Imaging the entire pathway (MRI head and neck down to T2 with MRA neck) may be necessary if further localization cannot be performed due to difficulties with hydroxyamphetamine availability.

Table 4-2. Guidelines for Ordering Imaging Studies in Ophthalmology

1. Decide whether CT or MRI is indicated. The MRI scan is superior to CT for most neuro-ophthalmic indications, but CT is superior to MRI for calcification, bone, acute hemorrhage, if an emergent scan is needed, or if the patient cannot undergo MRI.
2. Decide if contrast is needed. In most cases, contrast material should be ordered for both CT and MRI studies. Contrast may not be necessary in acute hemorrhage, thyroid eye disease, or trauma cases. Caution is necessary for both iodinated contrast and gadolinium contrast in patients with renal failure, and contrast may be contraindicated in these settings.
3. Topographically localize the lesion clinically ("where is the lesion"), define the differential diagnosis ("what is the lesion"), establish the urgency of the imaging request, and then order the best study tailored to the lesion location (e.g. head, orbit, or neck).
4. Order specific imaging sequences (e.g., fat suppression for orbital postcontrast study, fluid attenuation inversion recovery for white matter lesions, gradient recall echo for hemorrhage, diffusion-weighted imaging for stroke or posterior reversible encephalopathy syndrome) depending on clinical indication.
5. Order special imaging for specific vascular indications (e.g., MRA or CTA, MRV, CA). See Table 3–1 for catheter angiography, MRA, and CTA recommendations for third nerve palsy.
6. Call the radiologist if there is any doubt about localization, image study of choice, contrast selection, indications, or the final report.
7. If the imaging shows either no abnormality or an abnormality that does not match the clinical localization, then call the radiologist or, better yet, review the films directly with him or her. Ask the radiologist if the area of interest has been adequately imaged, if artifact might be obscuring the lesion, or if additional studies might show the lesion.
8. If the clinical picture suggests a specific lesion or localization and initial imaging is "normal," consider repeating the imaging with thinner slices and higher magnification of the area of interest, especially if the clinical signs and symptoms are progressive.
9. Recognize that the lack of an imaging abnormality does not exclude pathology.

Modified from Reference 54.
CA, conventional angiography; CT, computed tomography; CTA, computed tomography angiography; MRA, magnetic resonance angiography; MRI, magnetic resonance imaging; MRV, magnetic resonance venography.

4-3 EXAMINATION OF IMAGES

After review of the identifying and acquisition information, attention is turned to the images themselves. It is important to orient oneself to the plane of scanning. This may be done by examining the scout film, which shows the slices as sectioned by the computer. Axial and coronal images can be confused if one is not familiar with the area of the brain being imaged. Many software programs allow the user to measure the size of lesions with a virtual ruler and to check the location of a suspected lesion seen on multiple imaging planes. Reviewing the information on the scans requires experience. It is necessary to examine bone, soft tissue, blood vessels, and cerebrospinal fluid–containing structures to assess normality. Ideally, the prescribing clinician would review the imaging study directly with the interpreting radiologist to obtain the ideal combination of clinicoradiologic correlation.

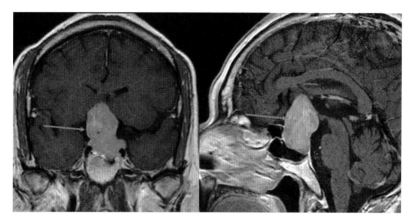

Figure 4-10. Coronal (*left*) and sagittal (*right*) postcontrast T1-weighted MR images showing heterogeneous enhancement in an intrasellar mass with suprasellar extension (arrows) and compression of the optic chiasm from below, consistent with a pituitary adenoma.

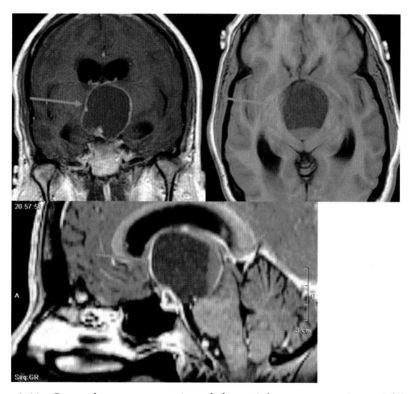

Figure 4-11. Coronal postcontrast (*top left*), axial precontrast (*top right*), and sagittal postcontrast (*bottom*) T1-weighted MR images demonstrating a cystic suprasellar mass (*arrows*) compressing the optic chiasm, consistent with a cranio-pharyngioma. The differential diagnosis could also include a Rathke cleft cyst and a cystic pituitary adenoma.

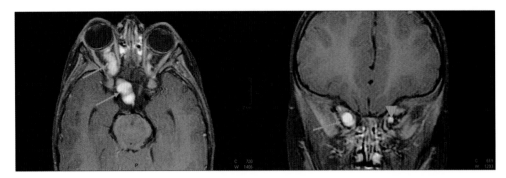

Figure 4-12. Axial (*left*) and coronal (*right*) postcontrast T1-weighted MR images with fat suppression demonstrating bilateral optic nerve enlargement and enhancement on the right (*arrows*) greater than on the left (*arrowhead*), consistent with bilateral optic nerve gliomas in a patient with neurofibromatosis type 1.

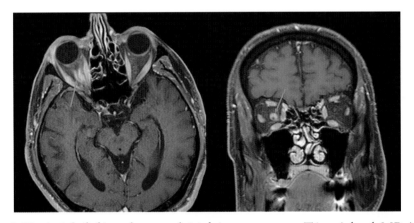

Figure 4-13. Axial (*left*) and coronal (*right*) postcontrast T1-weighted MR images with fat suppression demonstrating bright signal in the optic nerve sheath (*arrows*) surrounding the darker, nonenhancing optic nerve parenchyma, consistent with an optic nerve sheath meningioma. The differential diagnosis could also include optic perineuritis, sarcoidosis, and other infiltrative lesions such as metastases.

Summary

Ophthalmologists should be aware of the basics of magnetic resonance (MR) and computed tomography (CT) scanning. In general, MR imaging is superior to CT scanning for most intracranial neuro-ophthalmic indications. However, CT still has a role for assessment of acute hemorrhage, hydrocephalus, bone pathology, trauma, orbital disease, sinus disease, and thyroid eye disease and for evaluating patients unable to undergo an MR scan or in emergent situations. Neuro-ophthalmic indications and guidelines for choosing the most appropriate imaging modality are summarized in Table 4-1. In general, contrast material should be ordered for neuro-ophthalmic indications, unless there is a clear contraindication. Awareness of special MR sequences is needed as they may not be included in standard imaging protocols in some regions. These sequences include fat suppression, fluid-attenuated inversion recovery, gradient echo, and diffusion-weighted imaging. Ophthalmologists should also be aware of evolving techniques in vascular imaging (magnetic resonance angiography and computed tomography angiography) as they are reducing the need for catheter angiography in certain settings. Finally, functional imaging, such as positron-emission tomography, may be indicated in patients with normal structural neuroimaging studies or for the evaluation of underlying systemic inflammatory or neoplastic disorders that produce eye findings (e.g., paraneoplastic disease). Again, we stress the critical importance for the ordering ophthalmologist to provide the radiologist with the pertinent clinical findings, a useful differential diagnosis, and the suspected location of a lesion to obtain the best study and interpretation.

References

1. Juttler E, Fiebach JB, Schellinger PD. Diagnostic imaging for acute ischemic stroke management. *Expert Rev Med Devices*. 2006;3(1):113–126.
2. Barboriak DP. Imaging of brain tumors with diffusion-weighted and diffusion tensor MR imaging. *Magn Reson Imaging Clin North Am*. 2003;11(3):379–401.
3. Gregory DG, Pelak VS, Bennett JL. Diffusion-weighted magnetic resonance imaging and the evaluation of cortical blindness in preeclampsia. *Surv Ophthalmol*. 2003;48(6):647–650.
4. Kolb SJ, Costello F, Lee AG, et al. Distinguishing ischemic stroke from the stroke-like lesions of MELAS using apparent diffusion coefficient mapping. *J Neurol Sci*. 2003;216(1):11–15.
5. Romano A, Bozzao A, Bonamini M, et al. Diffusion-weighted MR imaging: clinical applications in neuroradiology. *Radiol Med (Torino)*. 2003;106(5–6):521–548.
6. Stadnik TW, Demaerel P, Luypaert RR, et al. Imaging tutorial: differential diagnosis of bright lesions on diffusion-weighted MR images. *RadioGraphics*. 2003;23(1):e7.
7. Valentini V, Gaudino S, Spagnolo P, et al. Diffusion and perfusion MR imaging. *Rays*. 2003;28(1):29–43.
8. Bammer R. Basic principles of diffusion-weighted imaging. *Eur J Radiol*. 2003;45(3):169–184.
9. Rovaris M, Rocca MA, Filippi M. Magnetic resonance-based techniques for the study and management of multiple sclerosis. *Br Med Bull*. 2003;65:133–144.
10. Rosen BR, Belliveau JW, Vevea JM, Brady TJ. Perfusion imaging with NMR contrast agents. *Magn Reson Med*. 1990;14(2):249–265.
11. Jansen O, Schellinger P, Fiebach J, et al. Early recanalisation in acute ischaemic stroke saves tissue at risk defined by MRI. *Lancet*. 1999;353(9169):2036–2037.
12. Wolf RL, Detre JA. Clinical neuroimaging using arterial spin-labeled perfusion magnetic resonance imaging. *Neurotherapeutics*. 2007;4(3):346–359.

13. Glenn LW. Innovations in neuroimaging of skull base pathology. *Otolaryngol Clin North Am*. 2005;38(4):613–629.

14. Lee AG, Hayman LA, Ross AW. Neuroimaging contrast agents in ophthalmology. *Surv Ophthalmol*. 2000;45(3):237–253.

15. US Food and Drug Administration. Information for Healthcare Professionals Gadolinium-Based Contrast Agents for Magnetic Resonance Imaging (marketed as Magnevist, MultiHance, Omniscan, OptiMARK, ProHance). Accessed 17 May 2010. Available from: http://www.fda.gov/Drugs/DrugSafety/PostmarketDrugSafety InformationforPatientsandProviders/ucm142884.htm

16. Buxton R. *Introduction to Functional Magnetic Resonance Imaging*. Cambridge, UK: Cambridge University Press; 2001.

17. Willinek WA, Kuhl CK. 3.0 T neuroimaging: technical considerations and clinical applications. *Neuroimag Clin North Am*. 2006;16(2):217–228, ix.

18. Lancaster JL, Glickman RD, Schulte AV. Strategies for 3-D visualization of ocular structures. *Neurosci Biobehav Rev*. 1993;17(4):451–458.

19. Udupa JK. Three-dimensional visualization and analysis methodologies: a current perspective. RadioGraphics 1999;19(3):783–806.

20. John NW, McCloy RF. Navigating and visualizing three-dimensional data sets. *Br J Radiol*. 2004;77(Spec No 2):S108–S113.

21. Wintermark M, Sesay M, Barbier E, et al. Comparative overview of brain perfusion imaging techniques. *J Neuroradiol*. 2005;32(5):294–314.

22. Eastwood JD, Lev MH, Wintermark M, et al. Correlation of early dynamic CT perfusion imaging with whole-brain MR diffusion and perfusion imaging in acute hemispheric stroke. *AJNR Am J Neuroradiol*. 2003;24(9):1869–1875.

23. Moustafa RR, Baron JC. Imaging the penumbra in acute stroke. *Curr Atheroscler Rep*. 2006;8(4):281–289.

24. Rumboldt Z, Al-Okaili R, Deveikis JP. Perfusion CT for head and neck tumors: pilot study. *AJNR Am J Neuroradiol*. 2005;26(5):1178–1185.

25. Brenner DJ, Hall EJ. Computed tomography: an increasing source of radiation exposure. *N Engl J Med*. 2007;357(22):2277–2284.

26. Amis ES Jr, Butler PF, Applegate KE, et al. American College of Radiology white paper on radiation dose in medicine. *J Am Coll Radiol*. 2007;4(5):272–284.

27. American College of Radiology. ACR Responds to NEJM Article on Radiation Risk Associated with CT Scans. Accessed 09 March 2010. Available from: http://www.acr.org/MainMenuCategories/media_room/FeaturedCategories/PressReleases/Archive/ACRRespondstoNEJMArticleonRadiationRiskAssociatedWithCTScans.aspx

28. Jacobson DM, Trobe JD. The emerging role of magnetic resonance angiography in the management of patients with third cranial nerve palsy. *Am J Ophthalmol*. 1999;128(1):94–96.

29. Lee AG, Hayman LA, Brazis PW. The evaluation of isolated third nerve palsy revisited: an update on the evolving role of magnetic resonance, computed tomography, and catheter angiography. *Surv Ophthalmol*. 2002;47(2):137–157.

30. Goldman JP. New techniques and applications for magnetic resonance angiography. *Mt Sinai J Med*. 2003;70(6):375–385.

31. Lee DH. Magnetic resonance angiography. *Adv Neurol*. 2003;92:43–52.

32. Tipper G, U-King-IM JM, Price SJ, et al. Detection and evaluation of intracranial aneurysms with 16-row multislice CT angiography. *Clin Radiol*. 2005;60(5):565–572.

33. Jacobson DM. Pupil involvement in patients with diabetes-associated oculomotor nerve palsy. *Arch Ophthalmol*. 1998;116(6):723–727.

34. Nederkoorn PJ, van der Graaf Y, Hunink MG. Duplex ultrasound and magnetic resonance angiography compared with digital subtraction angiography in carotid artery stenosis: a systematic review. *Stroke.* 2003;34(5):1324–1332.

35. Koelemay MJ, Nederkoorn PJ, Reitsma JB, Majoie CB. Systematic review of computed tomographic angiography for assessment of carotid artery disease. *Stroke.* 2004;35(10):2306–2312.

36. Renowden S. Cerebral venous sinus thrombosis. *Eur Radiol.* 2004;14(2):215–226.

37. Leach JL, Fortuna RB, Jones BV, Gaskill-Shipley MF. Imaging of cerebral venous thrombosis: current techniques, spectrum of findings, and diagnostic pitfalls. *RadioGraphics.* 2006;26(Suppl 1):S19–S41; discussion S2–S3.

38. Biousse V, Ameri A, Bousser MG. Isolated intracranial hypertension as the only sign of cerebral venous thrombosis. *Neurology.* 1999;53(7):1537–1542.

39. Friedman DI, Jacobson DM. Diagnostic criteria for idiopathic intracranial hypertension. *Neurology.* 2002;59(10):1492–1495.

40. King JO, Mitchell PJ, Thomson KR, Tress BM. Manometry combined with cervical puncture in idiopathic intracranial hypertension. *Neurology.* 2002;58(1):26–30.

41. Farb RI, Scott JN, Willinsky RA, et al. Intracranial venous system: gadolinium-enhanced three-dimensional MR venography with auto-triggered elliptic centric-ordered sequence: initial experience. *Radiology.* 2003;226(1):203–209.

42. Ozsvath RR, Casey SO, Lustrin ES, et al. Cerebral venography: comparison of CT and MR projection venography. *AJR Am J Roentgenol.* 1997;169(6):1699–1707.

43. Smith JK, Castillo M, Kwock L. MR spectroscopy of brain tumors. *Magn Reson Imaging Clin North Am.* 2003;11(3):415–429, v-vi.

44. Detre JA. Clinical applicability of functional MRI. *J Magn Reson Imaging.* 2006;23(6):808–815.

45. Dickerson BC. Advances in functional magnetic resonance imaging: technology and clinical applications. *Neurotherapeutics.* 2007;4(3):360–370.

46. Ettl A, Fischer-Klein C, Chemelli A, et al. Nuclear magnetic resonance spectroscopy. Principles and applications in neuroophthalmology. *Int Ophthalmol.* 1994;18(3):171–181.

47. Mathews D, Unwin DH. Quantitative cerebral blood flow imaging in a patient with the Heidenhain variant of Creutzfeldt-Jakob disease. *Clin Nucl Med.* 2001;26(9):770–773.

48. Moster ML, Galetta SL, Schatz NJ. Physiologic functional imaging in "functional" visual loss. *Surv Ophthalmol.* 1996;40(5):395–399.

49. Uoshima N, Karasuno T, Yagi T, et al. Late onset cyclosporine-induced cerebral blindness with abnormal SPECT imagings in a patient undergoing unrelated bone marrow transplantation. *Bone Marrow Transplant.* 2000;26(1):105–108.

50. Kurz-Levin MM, Landau K. A comparison of imaging techniques for diagnosing drusen of the optic nerve head. *Arch Ophthalmol.* 1999;117(8):1045–1049.

51. Peterson JJ, Bancroft LW, Kransdorf MJ. Wooden foreign bodies: imaging appearance. *AJR Am J Roentgenol.* 2002;178(3):557–562.

52. Yamashita K, Noguchi T, Mihara F, et al. An intraorbital wooden foreign body: description of a case and a variety of CT appearances. *Emerg Radiol.* 2007;14(1):41–43.

53. Wolintz RJ, Trobe JD, Cornblath WT, et al. Common errors in the use of magnetic resonance imaging for neuro-ophthalmic diagnosis. *Surv Ophthalmol.* 2000;45(2):107–114.

54. Lee AG, Brazis PW, Garrity JA, White M. Imaging for neuro-ophthalmic and orbital disease. *Am J Ophthalmol.* 2004;138(5):852–862.

55. Lee JH, Lee HK, Lee DH, et al. Neuroimaging strategies for three types of Horner syndrome with emphasis on anatomic location. *AJR Am J Roentgenol.* 2007;188(1): W74–W81.

56. Reede DL, Garcon E, Smoker WR, Kardon R. Horner's syndrome: clinical and radiographic evaluation. *Neuroimag Clin North Am.* 2008;18(2):369–385.

SUGGESTED READINGS

Atlas SW: *Magnetic Resonance Imaging of the Brain and Spine.* Philadelphia, PA: Lippincott Williams & Wilkins; 2009.

Edelman RR, Hesselink JR, Zlatkin MB, Crues JV: *Clinical Magnetic Resonance Imaging.* Philadelphia, PA: WB Saunders Co; 2005.

Harnsberger HR, Osborn AG, Ross JS, Macdonald AJ: *Diagnostic and Surgical Imaging Anatomy: Brain, Head and Neck, Spine.* Philadelphia, PA: Lippincott Williams & Wilkins; 2006.

Kretschmann H, Weinrich W: *Cranial Neuroimaging and Clinical Neuroanatomy: Magnetic Resonance Imaging and Computed Tomography.* New York, NY: Thieme; 2003.

Index

Note: Page references followed by "*f*" and "*t*" denote figures and tables, respectively.